Why this book matters

There is good news and bad news about diabetes.

The bad news is that type 2 diabetes is swamping the world like a tsunami and has become a leading cause of unnecessary death and disease. In 2015, the world will get its 400 millionth diabetic. In the time it takes to read this sentence, the world will get another three diabetics. And three more in the next 10 seconds. During this sentence, there will be one death from diabetes. And another in the following six seconds. The International Diabetes Federation (IDF) says the number of diabetics is rising by 10 million a year. We are on our way to 592 million diabetics within 20 years.

Diabetes: The New Epidemic provides the latest data and advice on managing and preventing diabetes and new recipes to help plan your diet, a critical factor in putting the brakes on diabetes.The earthquake that caused the diabetes tsunami in Western nations happened around the middle of the 20th century in the form of affluence, sedentary jobs, labour-saving devices, genetics and the introduction of processed foods on a large scale.

The waves began in wealthier countries like the United States and then spread to Europe, the Middle East and Australia. Asian countries were the next to get the wave as their middle classes emerged.

Soon the waves will overwhelm some health systems.

The good news is that individuals can easily avoid the wave by following a few simple life-saving rules. If you let the wave catch you, it is impossible to get off. One you have diabetes, you have it forever; the best you can hope for is to manage it or ride the wave through treacherous waters.

If you get diabetes and fail to manage it, you will die early. Or have a heart attack. Or lose your eyesight. Or lose your kidneys. Or have a stroke. Or have a leg amputated.

Most information about diabetes is either a disaster scenario or a fix-it guide that sounds too good to be true.

This book gives you the good news and the bad news in equal measure – 50 negatives, 50 positives and a page of contacts for more information. It's the 101 things you need to know to avoid diabetes death and add years to your life. Plus throughout the book there are more than 500 other facts and findings set out clearly and simply with practical ways to beat diabetes for a healthy life. Yes, Virginia, when it comes to living healthier and longer, there is a fountain of youth. And it is to be found within every one of us.

"Every human being is the author of his own health or disease."
Buddha

To my late father Maurice Conway Smith,
who died suddenly at 53 before many of the facts
in this book were known

Acknowledgments

The author is grateful for the printed and online resources of a number of leading centres for diabetes research and treatment in several countries. They include the World Health Organisation, the International Diabetes Federation, the American Diabetes Association, Diabetes Australia, Diabetes UK and Diabetes New Zealand. These organisations have been credited where appropriate. The author is also grateful to the publisher, Michael Wilkinson, for encouragement to amplify a message that is important for hundreds of millions of people around the world. Finally, thanks to Jess Lomas of Wilkinson Publishing for providing the recipes.

By the same author

Downsize Me, How to fight diabetes and a heart attack,
Wilkinson Publishing, Melbourne, 2007

An introductory word from Paul Zimmet

It is no surprise that Mike Smith's *Diabetes Guide* has been reprinted so soon after its initial publication. The book brings both good news and bad about the disorder which, in the period of three decades has moved from singular status to the fastest growing chronic disease epidemic in human history. And our knowledge about its treatment and prevention increases daily.

The bad news is that the epidemic continues its "rise and rise" and not only in developed nations but also in developing nations all around the globe. The association with obesity is noteworthy and the term to combine these two epidemics, diabesity, has been coined.

The good news is that finally there has been international recognition of the epidemic and, in 2006, in a unanimous resolution (almost unknown in history!), the United Nations General Assembly recognised the extent of the epidemic and called on all nations to address it.

Apart from the need for nations to undertake preventative action, Mike Smith's book gives plenty of personal tips on how to prevent type 2 diabetes, particularly for those who are at high risk.

Professor Paul Zimmet AO MD PhD FRACP FRCP FTSE

Professor Zimmet is a pre-eminent international expert on diabetes. He is head of the World Health Organisation's Collaborating Centre for the Epidemiology of Diabetes Mellitus. He was foundation director of the International Diabetes Institute in Australia and is currently Director of International Research at the Baker IDI Heart and Diabetes Institute in Melbourne.

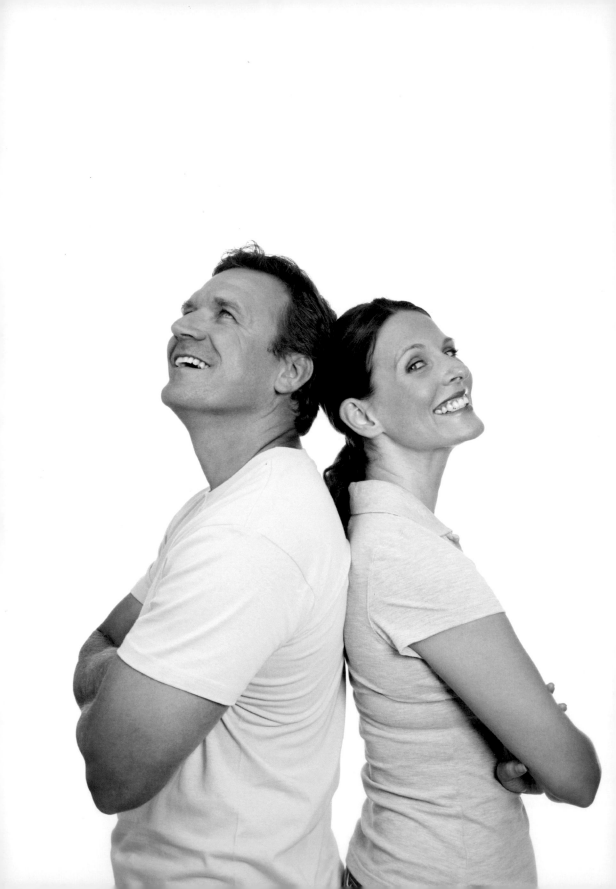

Contents

How I got diabetes and let it almost kill me

I should have known better. I should have recognised the symptoms: the constant thirst, frequent trips to the bathroom, bouts of tiredness and episodes of ravenous hunger.

I had been a medical journalist, writing about diabetes many times, including the need to watch for the tell-tale early symptoms.

But I was a bullet-proof young newspaper executive on a quick upward curve towards the editorship of *The Age* in Melbourne, Australia, rated by Columbia University and other independent judges at the time as one of the world's best newspapers.

Part of the newspaper's successful culture was working hard and playing hard, running the extra miles and never resting on the laurels of yesterday's story, which was today's history. For most editors, that meant leading by example; never asking your staff to do something you were not prepared to do yourself. The culture rewarded the young and the aggressive, the dogged and the doers.

Often that meant long shifts, skipped breakfasts, long lunches pickled in alcohol, snack food for dinner and then more alcohol late at night after the first editions had been put to bed. Sometimes there was an all-night card game before snatching a couple of hours sleep. It was a lifestyle common among professionals in many creative industries where young people were rewarded with rapid promotions if they worked hard and well enough.

Exercise was something for sportsmen and weekends were spent in recovery from five days of stress, smoke, alcohol, bad food and sleep deficits.

Had I acknowledged the symptoms, I may have been diagnosed before I developed full-blown type 2 diabetes at age 50. Even then, I could have avoided the worst consequences. My doctor said my diabetes was not yet severe and there was a good chance I could control it with diet and exercise.

I changed my habits. Slightly. Briefly. Before long I was back on the treadmill of bad food, alcohol, inactivity and stress. Not surprisingly, my diabetes worsened and my doctor prescribed medication to try to keep it under control. Next step, he warned, would be insulin. That sounded serious, I thought, and something to be avoided.

I mended my ways. I gave up cigarettes, stopped drinking, lost some weight and took up some regular exercise. It lasted a couple of years before I loosened the reins and let the professional and social whirlwinds take over again.

Before long, I was taking insulin twice a day. Insulin was a cinch, easy to administer from the modern injection pens. I learned to inject through my shirt at dinner tables and at the movies. It had a dramatic impact on my blood glucose levels and I could feel the difference almost immediately.

So effective was the insulin that it gave me confidence to chance my arm again on food and alcohol. Bad move. Dumb. Foolish. Stupid. Before long, I was on larger doses as my weight rose, and my blood sugar levels worsened. My blood pressure was up and I had unhealthy cholesterol levels. I was on a path to self-destruction. I was playing Russian roulette with a bullet in every chamber.

The heart attack came on the eleventh hour on May Day, 2006. It wasn't a classic Hollywood heart attack; most aren't. It began with some light sweating at a Monday morning client meeting, an annoyance I shrugged off as an after-effect of a hard weekend and the failure of the building's air conditioning to kick in efficiently at the start of the week.

By the time I was driving back to my own office, I had loosened my tie and opened the car window to let in some cool air. I felt a little heaviness across my chest; it wasn't pain and still I gave it little serious thought.

Fifteen minutes later, arriving at my office, walking from the car to the door was a bit of an effort. Walking up a dozen stairs felt almost painful and I was short of breath. At the top of the stairs, a wave of slight nausea swept over me. Now I realised I was in trouble. I called out to my secretary to drive me to the Melbourne's renowned Epworth Hospital, less than a mile away. In the car, it felt like a heavy weight was

sitting across my chest, like a weightlifter's bar. The feeling of nausea and dizziness swept across my body every 30 seconds or so and my mouth was watering. I was having a myocardial infarction, otherwise known as a heart attack, one of the most serious consequences for diabetics who do not manage their disease.

For many heart attack victims, the first symptom is sudden death. I was one of the lucky ones, enjoying good fortune I did not deserve. As I waited for the cardiologists to unblock me and insert two metal stents in my arteries, I remember seeing the faces of my wife, my children, my mother and my friends peering from above as they came to see whether I was going to live or die. At that moment, I decided that if I survived I would pay more respect to them by paying more respect to my health.

I survived. My heart made a complete recovery and I had been given a second chance. It was a second chance I would not squander. In less than two years, I lost 20kg and lowered my blood pressure and cholesterol to normal levels. The cigarettes and binge drinking were gone forever and my insulin dosage was reduced dramatically. I looked and felt years younger. One friend saw me on television and said he used to know me when I was older.

For me, it was a heart attack. For other diabetics, it might have been an amputation. Or kidney failure. Or blindness. These are some of the more serious consequences of the insidious disease of diabetes. The good news is that diabetes can be prevented. And even when it occurs, it can be managed. But diabetes must be taken seriously. Or you may die.

And as we shall see in the next chapter, diabetes is related to many other modern disease and lifestyle trends, which are shaping how hundreds of millions of people will live and die. Never before in history has the matter of life and death been more in the hands of the individual.

Diabetes and the big picture

At the beginning of the 20th century, the four main causes of death were pneumonia, tuberculosis, diarrhoea/enteritis and diphtheria. These were the so-called communicable diseases. More than 30 per cent of all deaths were children under five who were wiped out by the uncontrollable spread of these diseases.

The discovery that micro-organisms caused these infectious diseases and the development of antibiotics and vaccinations along with improved sanitation combined to reduce these deaths to a relative trickle in developed societies by the end of the century.

But they have been replaced by the rising death toll of non-communicable diseases, mostly lifestyle diseases. Much of it can be described as self-inflicted. Much of it is preventable.

These non-communicable diseases now account for 60 per cent of the 60 million deaths around the world each year. They include cardiovascular disease (mostly heart disease and stroke), diabetes and obesity. These three diseases have many things in common: they share common causes, they are all mostly preventable, the same preventative strategies apply to each, and they are all diseases of modern lifestyles.

One of the greatest strengths of our modern health systems is medical specialisation, which allows the aggressive pursuit of excellence in specific areas of medicine. It is also a weakness in that a silo mentality develops and experts are loathe to encroach into another specialty's field of expertise.

The result is that we have too few health experts who can not only see the bigger picture, but actively crusade on the world's biggest killer, the world's most expensive health problem, the mass suicide that will bankrupt health systems around the world in coming decades.

I have coined the term "cardiodiabesity" to help describe the triple whammy of cardiovascular disease, obesity and diabetes which is sweeping the world like a tsunami. Between them, they are killing 25 million people a year. That is more than any epidemic, famine or war has killed in such a short time in the history of the world. It is bigger than the annual toll of the Black Plague in the 14th century, more deaths than the 1918 flu epidemic, more annual deaths than any world war, more deaths than AIDS since the disease was first described and more deaths than from road accidents in the first 100 years after the invention of the motor car.

Cardiovascular disease is killing 18 million people a year, making it the number one killer and causing 30% of global deaths. Despite tremendous breakthroughs in medical and surgical techniques to treat cardiovascular disease and save lives, the incidence is rising so much that the World Health Organisation tips the death toll to rise by 30 per cent to 24 million by the year 2030.

Type 2 diabetes, what was once referred to as adult-onset diabetes, is the epidemic of the 21st century, rising at an astonishing rate in the past 20 years. There were more than 380 million diabetics in the world in 2014. That's more than 8 per cent of the world's adult population. And the number is projected to rise to 592 million by 2035. That's 10 per cent of the world's adult population; an average of 10 million new cases a year. The 2014 number of 380 million was more than 10 times the number a generation earlier in 1985 and double the number in 2000, only 12 years earlier.

Diabetes is killing 5.1 million people a year, according to the International Diabetes Federation. That's more than the annual death rates of AIDS, malaria and tuberculosis combined. They die from diabetic complications including heart disease, kidney disease, stroke and a host of other conditions. But that's only a part of the diabetic burden; millions more suffer major complications such as blindness and amputations. Diabetes attacks just about every cell and organ in the body. The cost of treating diabetes in 2013 was $US548 billion, about 11% of total health spending on adults, according to the IDF. Perhaps the most tragic part of the diabetes picture is that nearly half the world's 400 million diabetics do not yet know they have the disease and their body is being assaulted every day by the ravages of diabetes. And then there are another 320 million people with impaired glucose tolerance (IGT), many of whom will advance to diabetes unless they make changes or receive treatment.

Obesity rates have also risen at great speed. In 2006, the world passed a dubious milestone when the number of obese and overweight people surpassed the number of malnourished. Of the 1 billion people who were overweight, 300 million were clinically obese, exposing themselves to far greater risk of several deadly conditions including cardiovascular disease and diabetes. The World Health Organisation estimates that obesity is killing 2.8 million people a year and is a contributory factor in many more millions of deaths. One of the more alarming recent trends in diabetes and obesity is that the diseases are appearing in people much younger than a generation ago.

The three diseases that make up "cardiodiabesity" are linked by the modern lifestyle. We are less active in our occupations and daily lives. We eat more food and a much bigger proportion of it is processed rather than fresh.

The changing economy meant that many people switched from physical labour to office jobs. Rising affluence and the growth of cities meant that families bought more cars. Children stopped walking or cycling to school as the urban sprawl created greater distances to daily destinations. Children stayed inside with their televisions, computer games and video games instead of playing active games in the streets, parks or large backyards. Mothers started working and had less time to prepare home-cooked meals.

Even the developments of air conditioning and heating have been blamed for being part of the problem. Apparently we have lower appetites in extreme heat and expend more energy in extreme cold. Food supplies gradually shifted from local markets and stores to multinational industries. Food science provided preservatives and additives that extended the shelf life of food, which helped to bring down costs. Packaged food became much cheaper and therefore more attractive.

The big food companies knew that fat, sugar and salt were the most seductive taste sensations for human beings. Many packaged foods were loaded with these three addictions, packed with calories but short on goodness. They came in bigger and bigger packages, cleverly marketed and deviously priced to encourage the purchase of more rather than less.

A generation or two ago, family meals happened three times a day and anything in between was a treat. Today, the household refrigerator and pantry is open 24/7 and our shopping centres and workplaces are studded with convenience food outlets and machines. Eating and drinking is a round-the-clock activity.

The most dramatic increases in cardiovascular disease, obesity and diabetes have been in countries where the lifestyle and dietary changes have been most sudden, particularly China and India in recent years. Nearly 15% of the Chinese population is now overweight. The incidence of overweight children in China increased 28-fold in the 15 years to 2005 alongside a trebling of the percentage of food intake coming from animal sources in the 40 years to 2001, and the number of cars in China rising from six million to 20 million in the five years from 2000.

The numbers surrounding cardiodiabesity are chilling and horrifying. Anthropologists and historians in the future will wonder what we were thinking. They will note that for 100 years the human body gradually became taller with improvements in nutrition and then became wider as we switched to processed foods and swallowed too much of a good thing. They

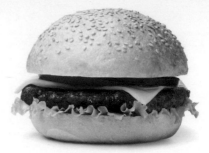

will notice how sports administrators at the beginning of the 21st century started installing wider seats as the average spectator's derriere grew, how hospitals started installing bigger beds for obese patients, how special ambulances were designed to carry grossly fat people and how some airlines began selling two seats to obese passengers.

Some of the most important scientific breakthroughs in this area have been the identification of risk factors and causes of the elements of cardiodiabesity. And therein lies the problem because the solutions rely not on magic bullets or miracle surgeries, but on personal action. One of the great social debates of the 21st century will be whether governments should educate, compel, reward, punish or encourage citizens and food companies to fix the modern world's greatest health problem, a problem that threatens to bankrupt health systems.

This book is principally about diabetes but recent studies have shown that the path towards preventing or managing diabetes is very similar to the path for preventing cardiovascular disease and obesity. A good diabetic diet and lifestyle is good for your heart and weight control.

The next step is to examine the principles of a lifestyle that gives you the best chance of avoiding the deadly troika in cardiodiabesity and not only adding many years to your life, but feeling and looking much healthier during your extra time.

Diabetes and depression – killer bedfellows

Diabetes and depression are two of the world's most common chronic illnesses. And they are remarkably intimate but lethal bedfellows.

In 2013, there were 370 million diabetics in the world. There were also 350 million people affected by depression, according to the World Federation for Mental Health in its report for World Mental Health Day on 10 October, 2012. And a substantial number of those people have both diseases.

Diabetes is one of the most pervasive diseases because it affects every cell in the body. Depression affects every aspect of human behaviour because it affects mind and mood. In millions of cases, they dance together to play havoc with people's lives.

There is an extraordinary link between the two diseases with evidence showing they are a consequence of and a contributor to each other. People with diabetes are at greater risk for depression and poor diabetes control can cause symptoms that look like depression. Someone with both diseases has a much greater chance of dying than someone with only one of the diseases. And diabetics with depression have more trouble following their treatment plans, have poorer control over their blood sugar and weight, have higher rates of diabetic complications, decreased quality of life, increased costs of health care, increased disability and more lost productivity.

More than 300 years ago, British physician Dr Thomas Willis was the first to link diabetes with depression when he suggested diabetes was the result of "sadness or long sorrow". Willis was also the man who added the word "mellitus" to the name of the disease, diabetes mellitus. The word "mellitus" is Latin for honey and Willis added the term to more precisely describe the sweet nature of the urine of people with diabetes, an observation that had been made for around 2000 years.

In the three centuries since Willis, researchers have firmly established the link between the two diseases, but they have still not proven why the link exists. There are two main theories. The first is that depression precedes type 2 diabetes and increases the risk of a person developing diabetes, because of hormonal changes which affect insulin resistance. The second is that depression in people with type 1 and type 2 diabetes results from the stresses of having a chronic disease and the constant self-management, which can lead to reduced quality of life and increased chances of depression.

Of course, both factors may be playing their part. Although drugs and insulin play an important part in diabetes management, the most important factors are self-managed care through diet, exercise, weight control, blood glucose monitoring and constant consultations with multiple medical practitioners. Sometimes a diabetic can have significant swings in their readings even when they are doing everything right and this can be frustrating, infuriating and perhaps even depressing.

People with depression often find it extremely difficult to motivate themselves to perform simple tasks, so the constant attention and dozens of tasks required to manage diabetes may seem an insurmountable hurdle for people with depression.

Depression can lead to poor lifestyle decisions, such as bad eating habits, lack of exercise, smoking and weight gain. These are all risk factors for diabetes. Depression affects the ability to perform tasks, communicate and think clearly, and this can prevent people from effectively managing their diabetes.

According to the American Diabetes Association (ADA), the stress of daily diabetes management can build. Diabetics may feel alone or set apart from their friends and families because of all the extra work. If diabetics face complications such as nerve damage, or if they have trouble keeping their blood sugar levels where they should be, they may feel they are losing control of their diabetes. Even tension between diabetics and their doctors may make the patients feel frustrated and sad.

Just like denial, says the ADA, depression can get patients into a vicious cycle. It can block good diabetes self-care. If patients are depressed and have no energy, chances are they will find such tasks as regular blood sugar

testing too much. If patients feel so anxious that they can't think straight, it will be hard to maintain a good diet. Patients may not feel like eating at all. And this affects blood sugar levels.

Measuring the link between diabetes and depression has produced differing results, depending on the type of diabetes and the type of population studied. Differences in defining depression have also clouded the research.

A major study published in the journal *Diabetes Care* in 2001 (Anderson et al, *The prevalence of comorbid depression in adults with diabetes*) considered 42 published studies that included 21,351 adults. They found that the prevalence of major depression in people with diabetes was 11% and the prevalence of clinically relevant depression was 31%.

A study published in 2009 by doctors at the Centres for Disease Control estimated that 45% of all diabetic patients had undiagnosed depression.

The International Diabetes Federation, in its *Diabetes Atlas Fourth Edition* in 2009, quoted studies which showed that depression was associated with a significant (60%) increase of type 2 diabetes, while type 2 diabetes was only associated with a moderate (15%) risk of depression.

Other studies have shown that complications of diabetes are greater among people with depression. These include eye problems, nerve damage and sexual dysfunction. People with both diseases also have higher rates of coronary heart disease. Katon et al in the US in 2008 published a study that showed diabetics with depression had a 36% to 38% increased risk of dying over a two-year period.

Egede et al in *Diabetes Care* in 2002 found that among diabetics, total health care spending was 4.5 times greater among men who were depressed.

So although the precise nature of the link is unclear, there is no doubt that diabetes and depression is a deadly and expensive combination.

Diabetics should be alert for symptoms of depression. These include sleeping too much or too little, lethargy or fatigue, feelings of sadness/anxiety/isolation, thoughts of hopelessness/harming yourself/suicide, trouble focussing or concentrating and not getting pleasure from pleasurable activities.

Having some anxiety, trouble sleeping or sadness after being diagnosed a diabetic may not indicate clinical depression. It might just be a temporary and natural reaction to being diagnosed and having to adjust your lifestyle and giving away some of the things you enjoyed. But persistent symptoms should be checked with a mental health practitioner.

I can remember many occasions when I began to have thoughts that managing my diabetes was becoming a little tiresome. I became sad or angry when my weight went up by half a kilogram after a week of a faultless diet and intense exercise. Maybe I got a bit depressed when my blood glucose levels spiked for no logical reason. Sometimes I would wonder about depression, particularly knowing that I had a brother, two sons and probably a father who suffered depression. But my feelings were usually fleeting and I was always fortified by the thought that I had gotten a second chance, which I probably didn't deserve, having survived a heart attack because I had not managed my diabetes. Life with diabetes can sometimes be a drag, but it sure beats the alternative. The lifestyle changes and medications I had taken in the seven years since my heart attack had given me the most

balanced and healthiest time of my life since my childhood. Managing diabetes was a small price to pay.

The ADA says if you are feeling symptoms of depression and have been feeling bad for two weeks or more, it is time to get help. Poor control of diabetes can cause symptoms that look like depression. During the day, high or low blood sugar levels may make you feel tired or anxious. The ADA says low blood sugar levels can also lead to hunger and eating too much. If you have low blood sugar at night, it could disturb your sleep. If you have high blood sugar at night, you may get up often to urinate and then feel tired during the day. Other physical causes of depression, says the ADA, can include alcohol or drug abuse, thyroid problems and side effects from some medications. Your doctor will be able to help you discover if a physical problem is the cause.

The ADA says if you and your doctor rule out physical causes, you may be referred to a specialist who can guide you through depression with counselling or antidepressant medications.

Diabetes and depression share many things. They are both annoying but can be managed and neither illness can keep you from accomplishing many goals and enjoying all your interests. Both can be helped by good food and exercise.

And for diabetics with depression, laughter may be the best medicine of all. And it's easy to swallow. Just forget the spoonful of sugar.

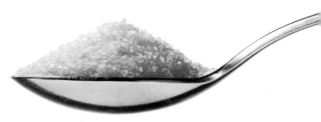

Beating diabetes – and getting your food plan ready

Ask any fairy godmother what is the most popular of anyone's three wishes and it's a fair bet that a long and healthy life would be at or near the top.

But cross-examine the Grim Reaper and he would tell you that more than half his harvest is people who have, in effect, caused their own deaths by adopting bad habits. The majority of those deaths are caused by cardiovascular disease, diabetes and obesity (cardiodiabesity).

Any person with a basic education knows that the key to weight control is diet and exercise. This is the starting point for preventing or managing the three diseases that make up the world's biggest killer.

So what gives? Everyone wants to stay healthy for a long life, they know how to achieve it but too many live like they have a death wish. Many people would be much better off if they treated themselves like they treat their pet dogs – plenty of exercise, fussy with food and occasional treats as rewards.

Earlier we discussed how changing work patterns and urbanisation have limited the amount of exercise we get in our daily routines. We also saw how our food industry changed the way we eat as our lives got busier. Sometimes it seems we are mainlining sugar, fat and salt as we feed our appetites for fast, convenient and tasty food cleverly marketed and packaged for high consumption.

A competing and confusing force is the weight-loss industry, which markets scores of so-called diets with examples of dramatic weight loss. These "diets" are mostly very restrictive and based on a narrow range of foods. It is little wonder that most people who go on these diets end up weighing more, even after an initial weight loss. It is too hard to maintain.

People have come to expect quick results because that it what they are promised. And it is often what is delivered in the early stages. But the diets are not sustainable because they are too narrow; they become tiresome and take too much enjoyment and variety out of one of life's great pleasures.

Similar forces are at work in the fitness industry. Too many people start with good intentions and excellent results, but the regimen is often too difficult to maintain.

So the first rule is to set realistic goals. Your diet and exercise strategies must be regarded as permanent and achievable changes, not temporary fitness "kicks" or diet "fads". It is far better to achieve gradual results over a long period than instant results which dissolve like fibreless junk food.

For most people it is a matter of calories/kilojoules IN versus calories/kilojoules OUT. The more calories/kilojoules you consume, the more you need to burn off. Burn more than you consume and your body will burn excess fat from your body. Consume more than you burn and your body will store energy in the form of fat. It's that simple.

With that in mind, there is a degree of choice about how to balance amounts of food against amounts of exercise. But no amount of exercise will compensate for daily overeating of unhealthy food. It takes a lot of exercise to burn off a few hundred calories or kilojoules which can be consumed in a moment. The smarter way is to limit food intake and then you need only a moderate exercise habit to achieve the energy balance or deficit.

Earlier in this book we noted how the diet for diabetics is now considered a good diet for weight control and good cardiovascular

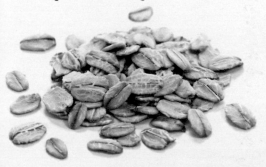

health. The principles of a good diabetic diet are to choose mainly carbohydrates, protein in moderation and foods high in fibre, avoiding saturated fats and foods high in fat as much as possible.

Carbohydrates are not just found in bread and potatoes. Other healthy foods rich in carbohydrates include beans, orchard fruit, sweet potatoes, sweet corn, lentils, high-fibre breakfast cereals and many crisp breads and cracker biscuits.

The first step is to invest some time investigating good choices about staple foods, the everyday foods that will always be in your shopping basket and pantry or refrigerator. By making good choices on these foods, you can reduce your intake of calories/kilojoules by the equivalent of many kilograms of body weight a year.

Find a brand of multigrain bread you can eat regularly. The fibre in grainy bread and some other carbohydrates – like beans, lentils and many orchard fruits – gives the food a low Glycaemic Index (GI), which makes your blood glucose levels rise more slowly than other foods.

Identify some favourite low-fat dairy foods. Visit the dairy section and check out the labels on low-fat margarines, milks and yoghurts with 1, 2 or 3% fat. Then choose the ones with the lowest sugar content. You should be able to find a margarine or butter substitute with less than 40% total fat and less than 10% saturated fat. Low or no-fat yoghurt is a good option for moistening pasta or vegetables when you ditch the sauces loaded with fat and sugar.

Stock up on canned baked beans, three and four-bean mixes, lentils, tuna and salmon. Check the labels and choose brands with the lower sugar and salt levels. These are all very healthy foods. Select an extra light olive oil for cooking, a much better option than oils with saturated or trans fats. Soy sauce, the salt-reduced variety, is a good flavouring for rice and vegetables.

Experiment with low-fat salad dressings and mayonnaises until you find some you like. Choose the low-fat products which are lower in salt and sugar. Do the same with jams and breakfast spreads.

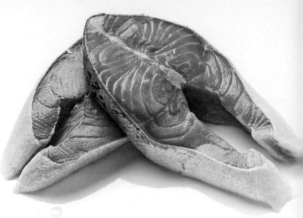

For me, the most difficult food to abandon was cheese. Low-fat cheeses (less than 5%) are not exactly a taste sensation but they can be a part of a healthy sandwich. Occasionally I will eat a small amount of very strong cheese to satisfy my real cheese cravings.

Choose an artificial sweetener (there are now some good natural options) if you need your drinks, breakfast cereals or other food sweetened.

The best low fat and sugar, high fibre breakfast cereals are the wheat biscuits under various brands and traditional or unrefined oats.

Finally, visit the spice rack and try some tasty spices to add some zest to your meals. There is no avoiding the fact that taking much of the fat, sugar and salt out of your food diminishes the taste, but the tastiness can be restored by using a wide range of spices. My favourites are pepper, mustard, curry, chili, cumin, dukkah and paprika. Cinnamon and nutmeg are useful with yoghurt or oats.

Once you have developed your buying habits for the staple foods, most of the rest of your diet is fresh foods including fruit, vegetables, fresh fish and lean meat. Deep sea fish like salmon and tuna are versatile foods high in healthy omega-3 oils. Choose white meats like chicken or other poultry and halve the calories/

kilojoules by taking off the skin. Use red meat sparingly and in small serves, trimming the fat. Eggs are fine occasionally.

Forget processed meats (too fatty and too salty). Keep pastries, pies, sweet biscuits, doughnuts, potato chips/crisps and confectionery off your shopping list. Unsalted nuts are okay in small quantities, with almonds the healthiest. Sugary drinks are a no-no; there are plenty of sugar-free options in the drinks section these days. And there is no healthier drink than water, which can help fill your stomach between meals, aid digestion and diminish your desire for food.

It's a reasonably tough regime. So now it's time to cut a bit of slack. There are 21 meals in a week, aim to get 19 of them right and give yourself two wild cards a week to take the foot off the pedal, perhaps when you are out for dinner or lunch and the best choices are not always possible. Don't overdo it, but enjoy the break.

Do the same with your exercise program. I give myself four wild cards a year to skip exercise when I may be sick, on the road or when the weather is just too bad to endure. Often after using a wild card I will make it up by doing two sessions the next day to keep myself in wild card credit. In the next chapter we will discuss exercise and its role in a good daily routine.

A day in the life - it starts with exercise

Like with your diet, the exercise program you choose should have achievable goals and be rigorous enough to provide health benefits.

Exercise burns calories (and therefore helps weight control) by increasing the body's metabolism to improve the efficiency of digestion and the conversion of food into energy. It also makes your body's insulin and diabetic medications more effective.

Exercise is like stoking the fire in your body's metabolism, making the furnace burn cleaner and more fiercely. This is good for circulation, and therefore your heart.

The exercise should be moderate at least. Moderate exercise should make you puff slightly and build up a light sweat. It should be easy to talk but not sing. Forty minutes of this type of exercise five times a week is enough for good heart health.

I chose brisk walking because I felt that was the kind of exercise I could maintain permanently. I never enjoyed running, could not be confident I could swim every day and cycling was dependent on a machine which may break down.

It suited me to do my exercise first thing in the morning, getting out of bed 90 minutes before the first of my other tasks for the day. For me, later in the day was too full of other duties and distractions which might interrupt my routine. Others may find the evenings a better option for exercise and there is a good argument for evening exercise as it promotes fast burning of the calories/kilojoules in the evening meal.

But for me the mornings were better. I liked the notion of getting my exercise credit in the bank before I did anything else. I also chose to walk seven days a week; for me it seemed easier to maintain the routine for seven days rather than waking up wondering whether it was a walking day or not. And I have my four "wild cards" a year, which I rarely use.

I began walking for 20 minutes a day, then 40, then an hour. I was surprised how easy it was to build up quickly. It is important to use good walking shoes and have comfortable clothing, including wet weather and cold weather gear. Choose an interesting walking path, perhaps through parks and along creeks or rivers rather than busy streets. Try to finish with a long or steep uphill stretch to lift your heart rate. Buy a device to listen to your favourite music, podcast or news. All of these tips help make the walk enjoyable rather than a chore. I'm a news and current affairs junkie, so I use the hour to get up to date on local, national and international news. I arrive home well informed – and ready for breakfast.

Breakfast is the easiest meal to get right with foods that should always be kept in the home.

People with diabetes or a pre-diabetic condition are encouraged to eat small meals with light snacks in between. This helps regulate blood glucose levels at more constant levels, avoiding the highs and lows commonly associated with diabetes.

The snacks should be low-fat, low-sugar and balanced. They can be taken mid-morning or mid-afternoon.

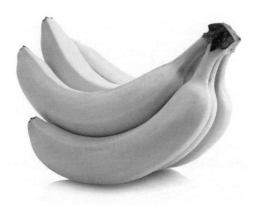

Breakfast
Small cup of traditional/unrefined oats
Fat-free milk
Artificial sweetener (optional)
Fresh fruit (with oats or separately)
One slice of wholegrain bread with low-fat margarine and low-sugar jam
Hot tea or coffee
Glass of water

Alternative breakfast
Two or three wheat biscuits
Fat-free milk
Honey to sweeten (optional)
Glass of freshly-squeezed fruit juice
One crumpet with low-fat margarine and yeast extract
Hot tea or coffee
Glass of water

Second alternative breakfast
One cup of low-fat, low-sugar muesli
Fat-free milk
Boiled egg
One slice of wholegrain bread
Hot tea or coffee
Non-sugar sweetener (optional)
Glass of water

Snack
One piece of orchard fruit
One or two dry biscuits
Water or sugar-free drink

Alternative snack
One fruit scone
Cup of tea or coffee

Second alternative snack
Two puffed rice cakes with low-fat hummus or tomato/onion salsa
Fruit juice

Third alternative snack
Small handful of nuts
Banana

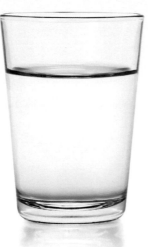

Lunch
Wholegrain roll with falafel or lean meat or low-fat cheese with salad or vegetables
Piece of fruit
Tea, water, sugarless drink or fresh fruit or vegetable juice

Alternative lunch
Bowl of soup – vegetable, corn or lentil with spices
Small wholegrain roll
One fruit scone or piece of fruit
Tea or sugar-free drink

Two-minute alternative lunch
Baked beans on one slice of wholegrain toast
Small side salad
Slice of banana cake or fruit cake
Tea or sugar-free drink

Snack time is a good cue to move around a bit whether at home or at work. Get up and walk around your home or office, perhaps up a flight of stairs or two. If you are going to a meeting or running an errand, take a walk. Park your car a little further from your destination. Walk to the second nearest train station or bus stop rather than the nearest. All this helps keep the body furnace burning.

Lunch is a meal that is easy to get right whether at home or work.

The evening meal is when the protein can be built up if breakfast and lunch have been short on protein.

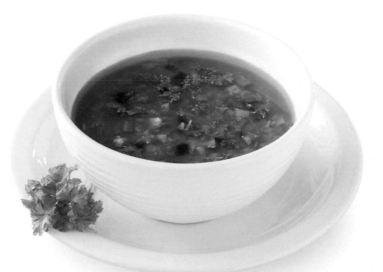

Dinner

Small to medium serve of grilled fresh fish
Two green or orange vegetables (steamed or roasted)
One potato (high GI)
One sweet potato (low GI)
Low-fat plain yoghurt and spices for moisture and taste
Fresh fruit salad or piece of whole fruit

Alternative dinner

Small to medium serve of skinless chicken or trimmed red meat
Vegetables/potatoes/plain yoghurt/spices (as above)
Low-fat fruit yoghurt
Fresh fruit salad

Second alternative dinner

Stir-fry vegetables with chicken or lean meat pieces
Salt-reduced soy sauce, spices and no-fat yoghurt to taste
Cup of Basmati or Doongara rice, boiled (both low GI)
Banana muffin with low-fat ice cream

Third alternative dinner

Bowl of wholemeal or high-fibre pasta
Sauce made of tomatoes, vegetables and sprinkled with parmesan
Small side bowl of three or four-bean mix
Fat-free or low-fat yoghurt

Two-minute alternative dinner

Salad with canned tuna or salmon and low-fat dressing and pepper
One slice wholegrain bread
Fat-free or low-fat yoghurt
Glass of water

Try to avoid snacking in the evening. Many people eat perfectly from breakfast to dinner then undo the good work by snacking on fatty and sugary foods at night in front of the television. This is the worst time of the day to increase your food intake because your body's metabolism is slowing down and is less able to process the calories/kilojoules. Avoid this trap by drinking water or trying food that is almost calorie-free such as salsa (home made with tomatoes, onion, chilli and pepper) or popcorn (without the butter or salt).

The next part of the book is the core section which tells you the 101 things you need to know about diabetes – the good news and the bad.

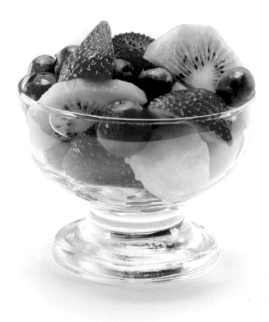

The 101 things you need to know about diabetes

Epidemic of the Century

Diabetes is the epidemic of the 21st century. Before the new century was 15 years old, the number of diabetics in the world topped 380 million. Noted international diabetes expert Professor Paul Zimmet has described it as perhaps the fastest-growing disease in human history.

The rate of increase was phenomenal. In 2005, the World Health Organisation predicted that the 300 million diabetics figure would be reached in 2025. Within five years, the diabetes tidal wave had swamped the estimate 15 years ahead of schedule. This was a ten-fold increase in less than 25 years. The number of diabetics in the world had doubled in 10 years. It affects more than 8% of the world's adult population. In a single generation, diabetes had become one of the world's most serious health problems and the new prediction from the International Diabetes Federation (IDF) was that there would be more than 592 million diabetics in the world by 2035.

The diabetes league table is topped by China (98.4 million) and India (65.1 million) but the highest rates of diabetes are in the Middle East and Pacific Islands.

Affluent western countries have big adult diabetes problems. In the United States in 2013, there were 24.4 million diabetics. In Australia, there were 1.65 million. In the United Kingdom, there were 3 million and in New Zealand there were 345,000 diabetics.

But the global data shows that an even bigger burden is borne by low and middle-income countries and diabetes is disproportionately affecting lower socio-economic groups, the disadvantaged and minorities in rich countries.

It's just about all preventable

The best news about the diabetes epidemic is that it's almost entirely preventable.

Just as the scourges of smallpox and other communicable diseases were wiped out by vaccines and antibiotics in the 20th century, the modern plague of diabetes can be eliminated in the 21st.

But diabetes is a much bigger challenge because it relies not on the ingenuity of a few scientist heroes, but the behaviour of whole populations around the world.

Human achievements in the past 100 years are astonishing; in transport, construction, communications, medicine, sport, literature and the arts. But our capacity for self-destruction is also formidable. In the second half of the 20th century, cigarette smoking was the biggest cause of preventable death until the message finally got through and smoking rates dropped to less than 20 per cent in advanced countries. Now obesity and its related conditions like diabetes represent the biggest cause of preventable death.

Type 2 diabetes makes up 85 per cent of the diabetes problem. In most cases, it is prevented by eating properly and exercising adequately. Simple as that. Diet and exercise can save millions of lives a year and untold billions in suffering and health costs. Simple as that. Yet the epidemic continues to grow because people do not seem prepared to change their lifestyle.

In the 22nd century, people will look back and ask "Whatever were they thinking?"

Diabetes is a big killer

Diabetes is not just an uncomfortable disease of older people, it is a major killer and one of the greatest causes of illness and death in most countries.

The IDF says 5.1 million adult deaths (20-79 age group) could be attributed to diabetes in 2013. That's more than 8.4% of all deaths in that age group. And it is a contributing factor to many more millions of deaths from cardiovascular disease, kidney failure and cancer.

The World Health Organisation says diabetes deaths are likely to increase by 50 per cent in the next 10 years in the absence of urgent action.

In the United States, there were 192,725 deaths attributable to diabetes in 2013. In Australia, the figure was 9,765 and in the United Kingdom 24,897. In New Zealand, the figure was 2,145. These numbers dwarf the annual tolls from motor car accidents in those countries.

In India, the IDF estimated that more than a million deaths could be attributed to diabetes in 2013 and the toll in China may be just as big after revised estimates of the rate of diabetes put the number of diabetics in China at 98.4 million.

Breakthroughs past and future

can help you beat diabetes

As we approach the 100th anniversary of insulin treatment, medical science may be on the verge of the next big breakthroughs for beating diabetes.

Before insulin was developed in the 1920s, most diabetics died young. They died before they developed the complications now commonly associated with the disease. Insulin saved their lives, but soon diabetics discovered that long exposure to the disease killed or damaged their kidneys, eyes, limbs and many other parts of their body. Eventually, many diabetics died from the disease.

From the 1950s, scientists developed a range of drugs to help fight diabetes and manage the complications. They learned more about the way diabetes eroded parts of the body and how this could be prevented or slowed with medicines, diet and exercise. The drugs have been continually improving in the decades since then and more drugs are developed each year. Within 10 years, there could be 50 different drugs available for diabetes, providing doctors with a large menu to tailor specific drug regimes for each patient according to particular symptoms. Newer drugs under development include hormones

that affect the brain's perceptions of hunger and fullness as well as the brain's capacity to regulate insulin production. At the Harvard Stem Cell Institute, doctors have found a hormone that increases by 30 times the rate of insulin production in the cells of mice.

The "Holy Grail" of diabetes research is the artificial pancreas, using an implantable device to measure blood sugar and release precise amounts of insulin required to regulate the levels. Elements of an artificial pancreas have been demonstrated as feasible in clinical trials, but the "Holy Grail" is still many years away from routine use.

Meanwhile, pancreas transplants are becoming a reality, with more than 30,000 done in the past 20 years. But these have been done in patients with advanced diabetes and they carry too many serious risks to be considered for routine treatment. There is also a shortage of donors.

Stomach surgery to staple the stomach into a smaller organ and removal of fat tissue is on the rise and there are many reports of diabetic patients requiring less or no insulin after this surgery. But it is a drastic and expensive option which is unlikely to become routine.

Casebook Nauru – diabolically diabetic

The tiny Pacific isle of Nauru is known as the world's smallest island nation. The 21-square kilometre rock sits 42 kilometres south of the equator. One of nature's blessings for Nauru was covering the island with bird droppings which gave rise to a lucrative phosphate industry and lasted until the early 1980s.

Later in the 1980s, Nauru was used by Australia as a detention centre for refugees.

Nauru is one of the fattest nations on Earth, with obesity rates of more than 90 per cent. And it has the highest rate of diabetes in the world at 30.9 per cent of adults, according to the International Diabetes Federation.

Nauru is a case study in how diabetes can engulf a country going through rapid cultural and social change.

Independence for Nauru in 1968 brought great wealth as the country took full control of the phosphate riches. For a period in the 1960s and 1970s, Nauru boasted the highest per capita income of any sovereign State in the world.

Amongst other things, the wealth brought a dramatic change in diet. People who once grazed on fish, coconuts and root vegetables were now eating imported Western foods laced with sugar and fat. In a culture that equated status with body size and food intake, the local population quickly became fatter and more diabetic. A popular snack, according to some reports, was a whole fried chicken washed down with a super-sized beaker of cola.

By the end of the 1980s, the phosphate had run out and the wealth of Nauru disappeared. But the legacy of obesity and diabetes remained.

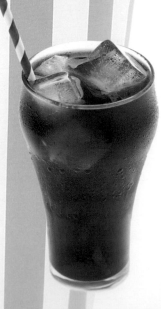

Know your disease – the simple guide

Diabetes is basically too much sugar (glucose) in the blood. The body needs glucose as its main source of energy and you make glucose from the carbohydrates you eat in bread, cereals, fruit, vegetables and legumes.

The glucose is carried around the body in the blood and then delivered to all the cells in the body to make organs work.

Insulin is critical for helping your body transfer glucose from the blood to the cells in your body. Insulin is a hormone made by the pancreas, a gland just below the stomach.

Insulin is like a key with a chemical message that opens the doors or channels for glucose to pass from the blood to the cells where the sugar fuels your body.

Diabetes happens when your body stops producing enough insulin or when your body cannot use insulin properly. Cells starve while glucose builds up in the blood.

For normal body function the sugar levels in the blood must be just right. In diabetics, too much sugar remains in your blood and this is what causes the problems with many parts of the body.

High Blood Sugar

OK

The analogy with petrol is not perfect, but it is like running your car on sugary or dirty petrol – the car does not run properly, things get blocked and the engine fails. Left untreated, your car dies.

This book is primarily concerned with type 2 diabetes, which makes up nearly 90 per cent of all diabetes. But there are two other types of diabetes; type 1 diabetes and gestational diabetes.

Nauru syndrome emerges around the world

A slower and more subtle form of "The Nauru Syndrome" has been washing over many parts of the world for more than 50 years. It has coincided with the rising tide of diabetes.

The post-war 1950s and 1960s brought rising affluence and with it came motor cars, labour-saving devices and the beginning of a big switch from physically demanding labour to desk jobs. Television arrived and changed our recreational activities from active to passive. Cities grew and so did the distances to jobs and schools. We drove instead of walked or cycled.

Food manufacturing underwent its own revolution, with processed foods replacing much fresh food because of its convenience and long shelf life. The fast food chains emerged with their relatively cheap and quick meal options.

Food manufacturers targeted our strongest taste buds – those that welcomed fat, sugar and salt. They super-sized their products and encouraged bulk buying.

Women joined the workforce in growing numbers and spent less time in the kitchen preparing food from fresh ingredients. For many families, eating became an all-day activity rather than a three-times-a-day necessity. We got fatter. And we got diabetes.

Compared to Western countries, China's economic growth and prosperity happened more quickly. And China's diabetes epidemic has emerged even more quickly than ours. In 2010, the International Diabetes Federation more than doubled the estimated number of diabetics in China from 43 million to more than 90 million.

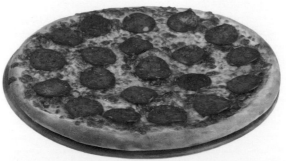

The other kinds of diabetes

Type 1 diabetes and gestational diabetes make up about 10 to 15 per cent of total cases of diabetes.

Type 1 was formerly known as insulin-dependent, juvenile or childhood-onset diabetes and is characterised by deficit insulin production and, unlike many cases of type 2 diabetes, requires daily administration of insulin. The insulin-producing cells in the pancreas are destroyed. Type 1 is not a lifestyle disease.

The symptoms of type 1 diabetes are similar to those of type 2 but are often more dramatic and sudden. The causes of type 1 diabetes are unknown and therefore it is not considered preventable. Some scientists believe it is an auto-immune disease where the pancreas is attacked by the body's own immune system. But it is possible that any auto-immune attack is prompted by another attack such as a virus or a poison in a foodstuff or the environment.

Type 1 diabetes usually occurs in children or young adults but many doctors have stopped calling it childhood diabetes because of the increase of type 2 diabetes amongst children.

Gestational diabetes is high blood glucose levels during pregnancy, possibly caused by hormonal changes. In many women it is easily controlled and treatment is usually limited to diet although insulin may be administered in more severe cases. It generally disappears after pregnancy, although women who have gestational diabetes are at a greater risk of developing type 2 diabetes.

Diabetes – the bankrupting cost

Diabetes is increasing so quickly and its impact so great that it threatens to send health systems broke and damage the economies of many countries.

The International Diabetes Federation estimates that diabetes accounts for 11 per cent of total adult health care expenditure in the world.

The total spending was estimated at $US348 billion in 2013 and this was expected to rise to more than $US627 billion by 2035.

An average of $US1,437 was be spent on every person with diabetes in the world in 2013.

But health care spending is only part of the cost. Other economic burdens include lost productivity, lost taxation revenue and foregone economic growth.

The Australian economic consulting firm Access Economics reported in 2006 that health system costs represented only 5 per cent of the total cost of diabetes. Of the estimated $A23.3 billion costs of diabetes in Australia in 2005, $A10.3 billion were in direct financial costs including carers, lost productivity and health system costs. The remaining $11.7 billion was an estimate of lost well-being in the form of pain and suffering and premature death.

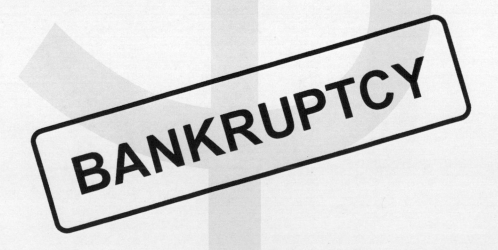

What causes type 2 diabetes?

What causes type 2 diabetes?

This is not a simple question. There is no single answer. But as more becomes known about the disease, it is becoming clearer that six main factors are involved:

- Obesity
- Poor diet
- Physical inactivity
- Strong family history of diabetes
- Ethnicity
- Age

The high-risk groups include people who are obese and have high blood pressure or heart disease. Ethnic groups including Asian, Middle East, Pacific and Aboriginal and Torres Strait Islander populations also appear at higher risk.

The more risk factors you have, the more likely diabetes becomes. Conversely, the more that people eliminate the risk factors they can control, at least to some extent (obesity, diet, physical activity), the lower the overall chances of developing diabetes or suffering severe complications once diabetes takes hold.

Health care rationing for diabetics

Millions of diabetics face health care rationing in the near future. Diabetes is one of a number of chronic diseases that are pushing up health care costs much faster than other costs incurred by governments.

More than two-thirds of health care spending on diabetes is spent on people aged 50 to 80 as they develop more complications from their disease. The ageing of the world's population will exacerbate the problem of diabetes spending.

These trends introduce a concept described euphemistically by health economists as allocation of scarce resources: health care rationing.

Diabetics have a few things working against them when doctors choose which patients should have priority. First, their condition means diabetics face more complications and therefore more risks associated with surgery. Second, diabetics develop more serious complications as they get older and doctors will increasingly have to decide between operating on a diabetic and operating on a healthier, younger person with better prospects.

Thirdly, some doctors may take the view that type 2 diabetics have a self-inflicted disease and therefore should have a lower priority. Already some surgeons are reluctant to operate on smokers or obese people. It is not such a huge step from here to imposing restrictions on treatment for diabetics who do little to manage their condition.

In New York, where the prevalence of diabetes is particularly high, some emergency ward doctors refer to recalcitrant diabetics as "shipwrecks" to be avoided in favour of more salvageable cases.

Don't beat yourself up – it's not all your fault

Diabetics should not feel guilty about developing the disease. Just as not all overweight people are lazy and slothful, nor are all diabetics guilty of neglecting their bodies or gluttony.

Indeed, there is mounting evidence that genetic and ethnic factors are significant for the development of diabetes. The US Center for Disease Control in Atlanta puts it at 60-40; 60 per cent caused by demographic factors (including genetics and ethnicity) and 40 per cent lifestyle.

Noted international diabetes authority Professor Paul Zimmet of Melbourne, Australia, says a major part of obesity is hereditary and children who have poor nutrition before birth are predisposed to type 2 diabetes, obesity, heart disease and even mental disorders.

Maternal diabetes and obesity shape the way the foetus responds, making it more likely that a child will develop obesity and diabetes.

Scientists also mention a human "thrifty gene" being partly responsible for diabetes and obesity. This gene enabled our ancestors to stockpile fat during times of plenty so they would not starve during times of shortages, famines and floods. In these modern days of 24-hour availability of food, the gene continues its work but there are no periods of shortages to work off the fat.

These genetic factors make it even more important that susceptible people act on the lifestyle factors that cause diabetes.

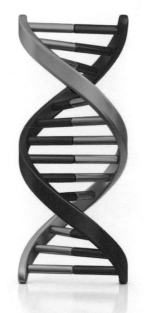

Suffer the children

Type 2 diabetes in the past was rare or unseen in children. The disease was commonly called adult-onset diabetes. But In recent years, more doctors are reporting type 2 diabetes in children and teenagers, especially in those who are obese.

The debilitating complications of diabetes usually take 10 or 20 years to develop. This means that a person who develops type 2 diabetes in childhood will be suffering the complications from their prime years of 30 to 40. This places an awesome burden on the individuals and the health system.

The increasing incidence of type 2 diabetes in children appears to be running parallel to increasing rates of childhood obesity. Scientists are also noticing higher rates in certain ethnic groups, similar to patterns in adults.

Some studies have indicated links with low birth weight, family history and exposure to gestational diabetes in the womb.

Some authors believe the incidence of type 2 diabetes in children is under-reported because many children do not complain of symptoms and some doctors misdiagnose the condition as type 1 diabetes, which has been historically associated with children.

The five-point plan – simple but not easy

There is a simple five-point plan to prevent, delay or manage type 2 diabetes. That does not mean it is easy but it's simple and capable of being easily understood by anyone.

The advice from numerous health and diabetes authorities boils down to a five-point plan:

- Achieve and maintain healthy body weight
- Be physically active – at least 30 minutes of regular moderate-intensity activity on most days. More is required for weight loss
- Eat a healthy diet of between three and five servings of fruit and vegetables a day and reduce sugar and saturated fats intake
- Avoid tobacco because it dramatically increases the risk of cardiovascular disease, especially amongst diabetics
- Get checked by a doctor regularly and have regular appointments with a number of health professionals if you develop diabetes

It is not easy. It requires permanent discipline and overcoming regular frustrations. But the rewards are great. This book will help you keep on track.

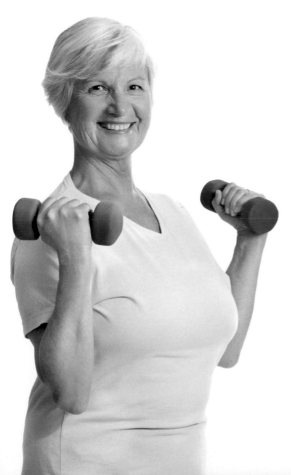

The rewards are fantastic

The five-point plan for diabetes provides everyone in developed countries with the chance to live longer and healthier. Following the plan costs no more than ignoring it, sometimes less, and there are no obligations to supernatural patrons or Middle East sorcerers.

Following the plan can prevent diabetes. If diabetes takes hold, the plan can manage the condition and delay or prevent the onset of serious complications, including death.

Diabetes can cost you anywhere between five and 20 years of life, depending on when it strikes. And preventing or managing diabetes can avoid many years of minor and major complications affecting almost every part of the body, from impotence to a heart attack.

And as a bonus, following the five-point plan can help fight a host of other diseases affecting a person's health and lifespan.

The upsides to following the five-point plan are unbelievably positive. And it's mostly up to individuals. As I said in my first book, *Downsize Me*: "Never before have such massive savings in medical death and injury been under the control of the patients themselves."

The symptoms

Diabetes groups in several countries list these common symptoms for type 2 diabetes:

- Being more thirsty than usual
- Feeling tired and lethargic
- Having cuts and skin infections that heal slowly
- Blurred vision
- Passing urine more frequently
- Tingling in feet or fingers

Some of these symptoms can pass unnoticed or persist for years without being recognised as serious. They can be passed off as general tiredness, getting old or a mild virus. People can become the proverbial frog in the school science experiment; oblivious to a gradual heating of the water until it begins to seriously damage or kill.

The tiredness occurs because the glucose is not getting into your cells to produce energy, as explained earlier in this book. Frequent urination occurs after glucose levels in your blood begin to rise and the body tries to get rid of the excess glucose by filtering it out through your urine. This makes you thirsty, so many people drink more sugary fluids, thereby setting in train a vicious circle.

Early recognition of these symptoms is a huge bonus for millions of people on their way to diabetes.

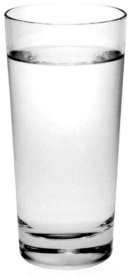

" (Diabetes) will have a major impact on the quality of life of hundreds of millions of people and their families, overwhelm the capability of many national health care systems and impact adversely upon the economy of those countries that are most in need of development. **"**

Nigel Unwin and Amanda Marlin, *Diabetes Action Now*, a joint initiative of the International Diabetes Federation and the WHO.

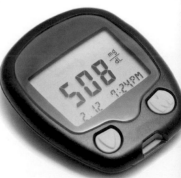

The bonus of early diagnosis

Doctors have identified two pre-diabetic conditions called impaired glucose tolerance (IGT) and impaired fasting glycaemia (IFG). Some experts estimate there are as many people with pre-diabetes as there are with full-blown diabetes. The big difference is that pre-diabetes conditions can be reversed if detected early enough. Diabetes, once it takes hold, is forever and cannot be cured; it can only be managed or controlled.

The other huge advantage of early treatment is that the more serious complications can be delayed or prevented. These complications often take 10 to 15 years to develop but good management can defer or prevent them.

If you believe you may have symptoms of diabetes, talk to your doctor and simple tests will reveal whether you have diabetes or a pre-diabetic condition.

> **We cannot afford to remain a bystander. It is time to give diabetes and other non-communicable diseases the attention they deserve.**

Dr Ala Alwan, Assistant Director-General of the World Health Organisation, 2010

A modern epidemic with a long history

Diabetes may be a modern epidemic, but its origins can be traced back 3,500 years. The first known reference was in 1552 BC when the Egyptian physician, Hesy-Ra, mentioned a rare disease that caused a patient to lose weight rapidly and urinate frequently. Already doctors were linking the condition to diet by recommending that those afflicted go on a diet of fruits, grains and honey to stifle the urination. Indian writings from the same era attributed the disease to overindulgence in food and drink.

Diabetes was given its name by the Greek physician Aretaeus (30-90 AD). He recorded an ailment with symptoms including constant thirst, excessive urination and loss of weight. He described it as 'the melting of flesh and limbs into urine'. He named the condition diabetes, meaning 'siphon' or 'a flowing through' of water. A century later, the Greek physician, Galen of Pergamum, mistakenly diagnosed diabetes as a kidney malfunction.

Around 1000 AD, the great Persian physician and philosopher Avicenna provided the first comprehensive description of the disease, including its remorseless clinical course and its many complications such a blindness and loss of libido.

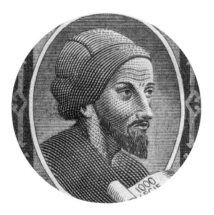

> " The high blood sugar due to type 2 diabetes, the high blood cholesterol and the high blood pressure now observed in younger and younger children constitute a national scandal. "

Marion Nestle, *Food Politics*,
University of California Press, 2007

The last 200 years makes it easier for today's diabetics

Early 19th century: Chemical tests to detect sugar in urine developed.

1869: German medical student Paul Langerhans described two sets of cells in the pancreas. Later one set of cells became known as the 'islets of Langerhans' because of their critical importance in the manufacture of insulin.

1870-71: French doctors notice that their diabetic patients seemed to improve during food rationing when Paris was under German attack, showing that some control over diabetes could be exercised by reducing calories.

Early 20th century: Fad diets for diabetes proliferate. They included the oatmeal diet, the milk diet, the rice cure, potato therapy and even the use of opium.

1920: Canadian doctor Frederick Banting and a colleague discovered insulin, for which he received the Nobel Prize.

1944: Standard insulin syringes developed, making diabetes management simpler and more uniform. Meanwhile, scientists establish links between diabetes and long-term kidney and eye problems.

1955: Oral drugs to reduce glucose levels introduced.

1959: Two types of diabetes identified – type 1 and type 2.

1960s: Home testing for sugar levels in urine helped people to manage their disease.

1966: First pancreas transplant occurred but failed to become a routine treatment.

1970: Blood glucose meters and insulin pumps developed.

1986: The insulin pen delivery system is introduced.

Early 21st century: Advances in stem cell therapy open up new possibilities for treatment.

> " **The life of a ten-year-old child who has type 2 diabetes will be, on average, between 17 and 26 years shorter than that of a healthy child.** "

Eric Schlosser and Charles Wilson, p214 *Chew on This*, Houghton Mifflin, Boston, 2006

Treatment – overview of a simple regime

Once you have diabetes you have it for life. The purpose of treatment is to control it and manage it, not to cure it. The objective is to keep your blood glucose levels as close to the non-diabetic range as possible, between 3.5 and 8mmol/L (millimoles per litre).

It is also best if you keep your levels as stable as possible, avoiding wild swings. Sometimes it can be like walking a tightrope, with a brief loss of control leading to an over-reaction and a problem in the opposite direction.

Milder forms of type 2 diabetes can be controlled with diet and exercise. But the usual progression of the disease is to require medication after a while and then insulin.

A person's blood glucose levels can vary according to time of day, timing of food intake, type of food intake, level of exercise, stress and other factors. Doctors are especially interested in your fasting level early in the day because that is when other factors are least likely to influence the reading.

Doctors may advise you to take several readings a day and learn what makes a difference. These readings are done with a pinprick blood test on a fingertip and analysis with an inexpensive computerised blood glucose meter available at most chemists.

These tests are extremely useful but no substitute for regular laboratory tests your doctor will order to get an accurate measurement of average blood glucose levels over the previous three months.

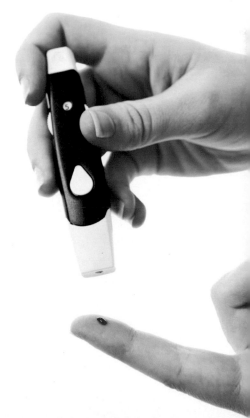

" A recent study in *The Journal of the American Medical Association* predicts that a child born in 2000 has a one-in-three chance of developing diabetes... today's children may turn out to be the first generation of Americans whose life expectancy will actually be shorter than that of their parents. "

Michael Pollan, *The Omnivore's Dilemma, a Natural History of Four Meals*, The Penguin Press, New York, 2006

Tablets can help your diet and exercise plan

Several drugs have been developed in the past 50 years to help patients manage their diabetes. Doctors may prescribe one or more medications if diet and exercise fail to control the diabetes.

If you begin taking tablets, it is important not to relax your diet and exercise programs. It is tempting to use the tablets as an excuse to ease off on diet and exercise, but that won't work. Maintaining a sensible diet and exercise plan can make the tablets more effective and delay the time when insulin may become necessary.

Diabetes tablets come from five main chemical families and they vary in dosage, potency and frequency of use. One of the most common is metformin, from the biguanide family. Metformin increases the sensitivity of the body's cells to insulin and reduces the amount of glucose produced by the liver. Taking metformin with meals limits minor side effects including stomach upset, rash or drowsiness.

Another family of drugs is the sulphonylureas. These include glicazide, glibenclamide, glipizide and glimepride. These increase your insulin production if you still have the capacity to make it. Side effects include stomach upset, skin rash, itching or headache. They should not be taken with some other kinds of drugs.

Other diabetes drugs include glitazones to reduce insulin resistance, mealtime glucose regulators to increase insulin production over a short period, and alpha-glucosidase inhibitors to slow absorption of carbohydrates.

Only your doctor will know the precise combination of drugs for your circumstances and history.

Insulin: an effective third stage

If tablets fail to control your diabetes, or if their impact diminishes, your doctor may prescribe insulin. It is injected because insulin cannot be made or work in tablet form.

There are many different types of insulin, but they all have the effect of lowering blood glucose. Compared to only a generation ago, today's insulins are very easy to administer; it is usually self-administered using a pen-type applicator with tiny needles that cause very little discomfort. Occasionally, I have injected through a cotton shirt at the dinner table or at a concert.

Your doctor will advise on how to administer the insulin, how to obtain and dispose of free needles and, most importantly, how much insulin to take and how frequently, depending on your medical needs and lifestyle.

The most important thing about blood glucose control is balance – too low is just as bad as too high. Some doctors say low is worse than high. The patient and the doctor need to discuss the timing of injections and meals. To maintain good glucose balance it may be necessary to have snacks between meals.

It is important to do regular pin-prick tests during the day so that you learn how your blood glucose is responding to food, tablets, exercise, stress and insulin. Only then, in consultation with your doctor, can you fine-tune your treatment and management to get the best possible results.

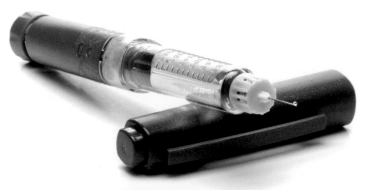

Dealing with the lows of diabetes

Blood glucose levels can go up or down during the day. The goal is to get them as stable as possible.

Levels are generally lower before meals, during or after exercise and in the middle of the night when there is a long time between meals. Higher glucose levels generally occur about two hours after meals and during stress. But everyone is different and diabetics should learn their patterns as completely as possible.

Low blood glucose is called hypoglycaemia, or 'hypo' for short. High blood glucose is called hyperglycaemia, or 'hyper' for short.

The symptoms of **hypos** appear quickly, over a period of a few minutes, and generally mean your blood glucose levels have slipped below 3.0mmol/L. This is easily checked on your blood glucose meter. Hypos usually happen only in people taking insulin.

Causes of hypos include too much insulin, lack of carbohydrate intake, excessive alcohol or excessive physical activity. Symptoms of a hypo are anxiousness or nervousness, palpitations or shakiness, hunger and disorientation progressing to confusion, mood change, belligerence and clumsiness. Prolonged symptoms can cause damage to the brain and nerves.

Diabetes groups advise diabetics with a hypo to first make sure they are in a safe place and stop operating a car or machinery. Have some quick-acting carbohydrates such as half a can of soft drink/juice OR three teaspoons of sugar or honey OR six or seven jelly beans. Wait for 10 to 15 minutes and repeat the dose of quick-acting carbohydrate if blood glucose levels do not rise. Symptoms should ebb quickly; if not, make sure an ambulance is called.

"How bad is the diabetes epidemic? There are several ways of telling. One might be how many different occurrences in a 24-hour period....so, 4100 people diagnosed with diabetes (in America), 230 amputations in people with diabetes, 120 people who enter end-stage kidney disease programs and 55 people will go blind. That's going to happen every day, on the weekends and on the Fourth of July. That's diabetes."

Dr Frank Vinicor, associate director of Public Health Practice at the US Centre for Disease Control, Atlanta, in *New York Times*, 9 January 2006

And managing the highs

Hypers happen when the blood glucose levels are too high, sometimes higher than 15mmol/L. A hyper comes more gradually than a hypo and can sometimes take days.

Possible causes of a hyper may be not enough insulin, too much food, an illness or infection and stress.

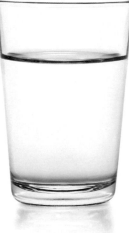

Symptoms include excessive thirst, passing large volumes of urine, dramatic weight loss, lack of energy over several days and progression to nausea and vomiting, abdominal pains, sweet smell on the breath, drowsiness and eventually unconsciousness in the worst cases.

The symptoms can usually be alleviated with more than the usual dose of insulin. Diabetics should talk to their doctor about having some fast-acting insulin on hand and drink plenty of water or other sugar-free fluid to compensate for the frequent urination. Seek medical treatment if the symptoms worsen.

Why exercise is so important

A kilogram of human body fat is about the size of a running shoe or medium loaf of bread. Unlike the red colour of fresh meat in your butcher's window, human fat is a sickly yellow colour and contains nearly 29,000 kilojoules (about 7000 calories), which is the equivalent of one Big Mac, a service of fries and a medium coke every day for a week.

A person who is 10kg overweight has the equivalent of ten of these slabs of death strapped to his or her body. It is difficult to think of a more destructive substance on earth, with the possible exception of tobacco. Fat prevents the insulin in your body doing its job properly. It increases your blood pressure and cholesterol, thereby increasing your risk of heart attack. It makes you look and feel bad.

Weight loss is a top priority for people trying to prevent or manage diabetes. Losing weight is a simple matter of burning more calories than you consume. We will deal with calories IN later in this book. Calories OUT is all a matter of burning them up with physical activity. Losing weight is not the only benefit of physical activity. It also helps the insulin in your body work better for 12 to 24 hours after exercise. It makes you look and feel better.

Physical activity helps weight loss in two ways. It burns calories and it raises your metabolic rate, which means your body burns more calories even when resting. Losing even a small amount of weight will help you control your blood glucose levels.

Half an hour a day of walking can halve the risk of developing diabetes, heart disease and high blood pressure, according to studies quoted by the British Medical Journal. Various studies show it is also beneficial for psychological and mental health.

When it comes to exercise, walking can be enough

The more exercise you can do, the better. But hundreds of studies have shown that the simple act of walking can improve diabetic and cardiac health.

If you can build up to more intense activity, that's fine. But walking is enough if you can build up to doing it briskly and for a minimum of five days a week for 40 minutes or more.

The benefits of exercise are immediate. You start to reduce your risks from the first step and the first calorie burned. Your exercise plan should be regarded as a permanent lifestyle change, not a temporary repair job. So choose an exercise plan that is realistic and one you can maintain.

When walking, you should move fast enough to puff a little, but not enough to prevent you participating in a conversation. You may have a very light sweat. This is the minimum effort required. If necessary, you can break it into two 20-minute sessions. Younger people should aim to do more.

Accept that walking is a permanent part of your routine, every day. Give yourself a day off on your birthday and Christmas Day.

Allow yourself three other 'wild card' days during the year. Choose cycling, swimming, gymnasium work or running if you prefer, but remember the relatively easy task of brisk walking is enough for good diabetic and cardiac health.

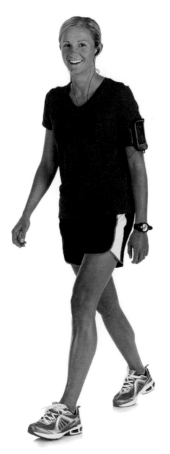

"Life expectancy usually decreases because there's a plague or a massive economic trauma. In this case, we will see a decline in life expectancy due to a chronic condition."

Mr Peter Muennig, assistant professor of Health Policy and Management at Columbia University, New York, *ibid*

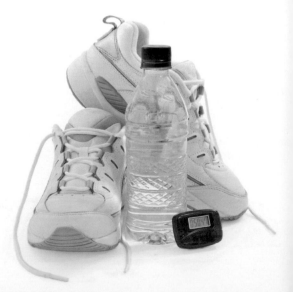

Ten tips for walking yourself to a longer life

1. Lock it into your routine at a particular time of day that is least likely to be disturbed. I prefer early in the morning because it gives me a head start for the day, making me feel fitter and more alert for the rest of the day's activities.

2. Don't rely on a walking buddy unless it is your partner, your dog or someone equally reliable and loyal.

3. Walk somewhere interesting and enjoyable. Trails or parkland provide a much more enjoyable experience than along streets with traffic and it will help you maintain your routine. If there is nowhere interesting near your home, drive or cycle to somewhere else to begin your walk.

4. Eat your breakfast before your walk, especially if you are on medication or insulin for diabetes.

5. Make sure you have a waterproof coat/jacket, scarf and gloves for cold or wet mornings. Do not allow the weather to interrupt your walk, unless it is extreme.

6. Keep your walking gear ready and near your bedside, in sight when you wake up. Make walking the first thing you consider when you wake up.

7. Use an iPod or radio to listen to music or news during your walk.

8. Plan a pleasant destination where you complete your walk or pause at the halfway mark. It may be a café for a hot drink or a place you can buy a newspaper or just a pleasant view.

9. Regard your walk as something to enjoy rather than suffer. The walking makes you healthier, and makes you look and feel better. Treat it like a friend, not a pain.

10. Vary your route every now and again to help you maintain interest.

" Imagine if kids were showing up at emergency rooms in cardiac arrest. Frankly, I think that's the next big thing. It's that dramatic. If diabetes doesn't respect age, why should coronary disease? Lord knows, I hope this never happens. But this is what keeps me up at night. "

Dr David L. Katz, director of the Prevention Research Centre at the Yale University School of Medicine, *ibid*

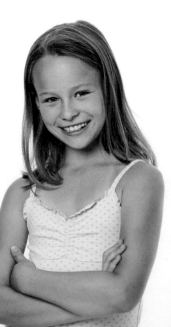

Turning on the after-burners

As we have discussed, there are enormous benefits to be gained with an exercise program based on 40 minutes of walking five days a week.

People capable of doing more can achieve even greater benefits. Diabetics and people with a heart disorder must consult their doctor about a more vigorous exercise program. It is remarkable how regular exercise can quickly allow your body to do more and more.

I decided to step up my exercise in the gymnasium. I was persuaded by the argument that converting some body fat to muscle would increase my body's capacity to burn fat. I realised that this would need to be a long-term commitment because unused muscles can quickly turn back to fat.

I had no desire to be a 'Mr Universe' but the notion of toning up in a gym where the priority was fitness and weight loss – rather than preening – was appealing. At a reputable gym, staff can design a gentle program for diabetics and heart patients. Remember to discuss it with your doctor.

My first session involved about 10 minutes of walking on a treadmill, about 15 squats, lifting a mere 15 kilograms on a bench press and some similarly gentle exercises for my arms, legs and abdomen. I learned how the machines worked and was taught the proper techniques for each machine. After my first two visits, I was on my own for a month or so, after which my program was reviewed and refreshed with different exercises. With each visit, you are encouraged to try to lift a bit more weight or do more repetitions.

If gymnasiums are not your things, you can build up your exercise program with more walking, running, swimming or cycling... but the basic walking program is enough if your weight is under control.

Three myths about diabetes

Myth 1: Diabetes is not that serious a disease

Fact: Diabetes causes more deaths each year than breast cancer and AIDS combined. Two out of three people with diabetes die from heart disease or stroke.

Myth 2: If you are overweight or obese, you will eventually develop type 2 diabetes

Fact: Being overweight is a risk factor for developing the disease but other risk factors such as family history, ethnicity and age also play a role. Unfortunately, too many people disregard the other risk factors and think that weight is the only risk factor for type 2 diabetes. Most overweight people never develop type 2 diabetes, and many people with type 2 diabetes are at a normal weight or only moderately overweight.

Myth 3: Eating too much sugar causes diabetes

Fact: It does not. Type 1 diabetes is caused by genetics and unknown factors that trigger the disease. Type 2 diabetes is caused by genetics and lifestyle factors. Being overweight does increase your risk of developing type 2 diabetes, and a diet high in calories, whether from sugar or from fat, can contribute to weight gain. If you have a history of diabetes in your family, eating a healthy meal plan and regular exercise are recommended to manage your weight.

Source: American Diabetes Association

Four more myths about diabetes

Myth 4: Diabetics should eat special diabetic foods

Fact: A healthy meal plan for people with diabetes is generally the same as a healthy diet for anyone – low in fat (especially saturated or trans fats), moderate in salt and sugar, with meals based on wholegrain foods, vegetables and fruit. Diabetic and 'dietetic' foods generally offer no special benefit. Most of them still raise blood glucose levels, are usually more expensive and can also have a laxative effect if they contain sugar alcohols.

Myth 5: If you have diabetes, you should only eat small amounts of starchy foods like bread, potatoes and pasta

Fact: Starchy foods are part of a healthy food plan. What is important is the portion size. Wholegrain breads, cereals, pasta, rice and starchy vegetables like potatoes, yams, peas and corn can be included in your meals and snacks. The key is portions. For most people with diabetes, having 3-4 servings of carbohydrate-containing foods is about right. Wholegrain starchy foods are also a good source of fibre, which helps keep your gut healthy.

Myth 6: People with diabetes can't eat sweets or chocolate

Fact: If eaten as part of a healthy meal plan, or combined with exercise, sweets and desserts can be eaten by people with diabetes. They are no more 'off limits' to people with diabetes than they are for people without diabetes.

Myth 7: You can catch diabetes from someone else

Fact: Although we don't know exactly why some people develop diabetes, we know diabetes is not contagious. It can't be caught like a cold or flu. There seems to be a genetic link in diabetes, particularly in type 2 diabetes. Lifestyle factors also play a part.

Source: American Diabetes Association

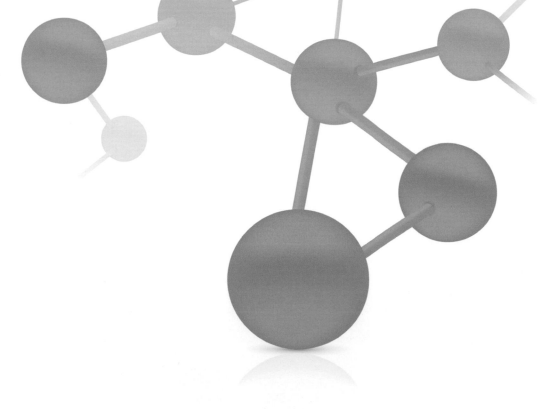

" Genetics may load the cannon but human behaviour pulls the trigger. **"**

Dr Frank Vinicor, US Centre for Disease Control, *ibid*

And a final three myths about diabetes

Myth 8: People with diabetes are more likely to get colds and other illnesses

Fact: You are no more likely to get a cold or another infectious illness if you have diabetes. However, people with diabetes are advised to get flu shots. This is because any illness can make diabetes more difficult to control, and people with diabetes who do get the flu are more likely than others to go on to develop serious complications.

Myth 9: If you have type 2 diabetes and your doctor says you need to start using insulin, it means you're failing to take care of your diabetes properly

Fact: For most people, type 2 diabetes is a progressive disease. When first diagnosed, many people with type 2 diabetes can keep their blood glucose at a healthy level with oral medications. But over time, the body gradually produces less and less of its own insulin and eventually oral medications may not be enough to keep blood glucose levels normal. Using insulin to get blood glucose levels to a healthy level is a good thing, not a bad one.

Myth 10: Fruit is a healthy food. Therefore, it is OK to eat as much of it as you wish

Fact: Fruit is a healthy food. It contains fibre and lots of vitamins and minerals. Because fruits contain carbohydrates, they need to be included in your meal plan. Many fruits contain high levels of sugar, which increases your kilojoule-calorie intake, so be careful not to eat too much fruit. Talk to your dietician about the amount, frequency and type of fruit you should eat.

Source: American Diabetes Association

Diabetes kills your heart

Between half and two-thirds of people with type 2 diabetes die of cardiovascular disease (heart attack or stroke).

Diabetics are three times more likely to have high blood pressure, obesity or elevated levels of blood fats such as cholesterol and lipids. This causes a build-up of fatty material in the blood vessels, which is called atherosclerosis. Diabetics are six times more likely than healthy people to develop atherosclerosis.

The atherosclerosis restricts blood flow, which can lead to blockages of blood vessels supplying your heart and brain. This is what causes the heart attack or stroke.

Cardiovascular disease is the leading cause of death in the world.

Love your heart and save it

Diabetics can reduce their risk of cardiovascular disease by taking effective medication and following simple control measures.

Apart from the normal diet and lifestyle rules for diabetics, there are a number of extremely effective drugs to combat the cardiovascular risks.

It is important for diabetics to have their cholesterol and blood pressure measured often so doctors can prescribe the appropriate drugs.

Losing weight and increasing physical activity will help lower blood pressure and blood fat levels. This will help your body respond better to the insulin you produce.

It is important not to smoke because smokers have double the risk of cardiovascular disease. Add that to the increased risk caused by diabetes and there is a recipe for disaster. My doctor describes smoking amongst diabetics as like adding petrol to a fire.

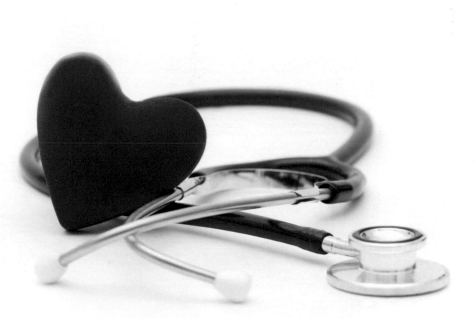

High stakes for your kidneys

Diabetes is the leading cause of kidney failure among adults in many countries. In Australia, for instance, diabetes is responsible for 33 per cent of new cases of kidney failure.

The diabetic damage to the kidney is known as nephropathy, from the *Greek nephros*, for kidney. It is caused by high blood glucose levels, high blood pressure and possibly high blood fat levels commonly seen in diabetics. People with diabetes are also more likely to develop urinary tract infections which can damage the kidney. Diabetes attacks the small blood vessels leading to the filtering system of the organ or within the filtering system itself.

For many years, there may be no pain or symptoms. Physical examination will not pick it up. Patients can lose up to 90 per cent of kidney function before symptoms appear.

Patients with kidney failure face years of dialysis in hospitals or their homes to flush their kidneys – if they are lucky. The success rate of kidney transplantation is high, but there are not enough donors. Most people with chronic kidney disease will die from cardiovascular causes before dialysis or transplantation.

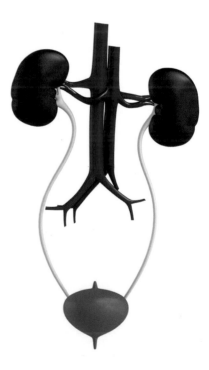

Use your kidneys and save them

Diabetic damage to the kidneys can be detected early through a simple laboratory urine test which measures how fast the kidneys are leaking a protein called albumin into the urine.

Doctors can prescribe high blood pressure medications called ACE inhibitors and Angiotensin Receptor Antagonists to help protect your kidneys from further diabetic damage.

Diabetics should make sure they have a urine test and kidney function test each year. At the first sign of a bladder or kidney infection, call your doctor.

And maintain your strategies for general diabetes control – diet, exercise and medications.

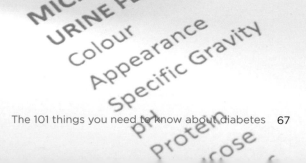

Diabetics can lose their legs

Amputees will become a much more common sight on the streets and elsewhere as the diabetes epidemic matures.

The most serious complications of diabetes seem to develop 10 to 15 years after onset among sufferers who do not do enough to control their disease. The world is now approaching the period of 10 to 15 years after the first dramatic surge in diabetes.

In the US, Dr Frank Vinicor of the Centre for Disease Control in Atlanta recently estimated that there were 230 diabetic amputations a day in the US. Many diabetics have multiple amputations, beginning with a small toe and gradually moving up the limb until the leg is gone. About 70 per cent of amputees die within five years.

Amputation is the final treatment for blood vessel blockage in the legs, known as peripheral vascular disease. The first symptoms are usually pain in one or both calf muscles after walking. Later, there could be ulcers appearing on the toes and feet. Then gangrene may develop.

Sometimes the blood vessels can be unblocked or bypassed through surgery. But surgery is often impossible because the blood vessels are so small.

Diabetics carry a risk of amputation that may be more than 25 times greater than among non-diabetics.

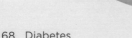

How to save your legs

Most diabetic-related amputations are preventable with scrupulous care.

The first rule for managing peripheral vascular disease is to follow the general principles of diabetes management with good diet, adequate physical activity and weight control as well as medically supervised drug treatment where appropriate.

Here are some other tips:

- See a podiatrist for a routine check every six months
- Wash your feet every day and dry them properly, especially between the toes
- Inspect your feet every day for cuts, abrasions, change of colour or swelling. Report changes to your doctor
- Check your shoes for rough edges or foreign material which might break your skin
- Always wear footwear inside and outside the house
- Buy a pair of "diabetic socks" from your local diabetes organisation for use during long periods of travel or sitting

If you are a smoker, giving up will give you the biggest benefit for peripheral vascular disease.

Risk to eyesight is plain to see

Diabetes is the major cause of blindness in people under 60.

The most common form of diabetic eye damage is retinopathy, where the small blood vessels in the back of the eye are damaged. This may cause a loss of vision due to an obstruction, bleed or leak.

The raised blood glucose levels and raised blood pressure in diabetics can cause blood vessels in the retina to become weak and prone to bleeding. Your body tries to compensate and grows more blood vessels, but these are also weak and prone to bleeding.

About one in three people with diabetes has some evidence of retinopathy, but it usually takes years before the damage causes blindness or even serious loss of vision.

Another common cause of eye damage is cataract, which is an opaqueness or clouding of the eyes.

According to the World Health Organisation, about 2 per cent of diabetics become blind after 15 years with the disease and about 10 per cent develop severe visual impairment.

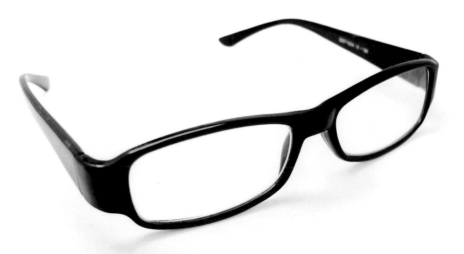

And the good news is also plain to see

The good news is that the rate of blindness caused by diabetes is falling. This is mostly because of improved treatments such as laser surgery and other procedures. But there are still millions of people who suffer diabetic eye damage and blindness unnecessarily.

It is vital that diabetics have their eyes checked by an optometrist ophthalmologist every one or two years. Check with your doctor how frequently you should have a check.

Appropriate treatment can halt the damage and loss of vision. And the best treatment is prevention by controlling your diabetes and blood pressure through diet, exercise and medication.

Nerve damage, diarrhoea and other unpleasantness

Nerve damage, or neuropathy, affects up to 50 per cent of people with diabetes. It is caused by high levels of glucose in the blood. It can also be caused or exacerbated by excessive alcohol consumption.

Many different problems can occur because of the nerve damage. Common symptoms are tingling, pain, numbness or weakness in the feet and hands. Nerve damage in the feet can combine with peripheral vascular disease, common in diabetics, to cause problems leading to amputations.

Nerve damage in the legs and feet can lead to a loss of sensation in the feet, leading to accidental damage because the person cannot feel any pain.

People with nerve damage can also miss the early symptoms of hyperglycaemia, which may occur without warning and cause episodes of convulsions, confusion or coma.

Nerve damage can also extend to the trunk of the body. In men it can cause sexual dysfunction.

Nerve damage to the abdomen can paralyse the valve at the bottom of the stomach, leading to vomiting. This can also delay the passing of food out of the stomach, which in turn can produce big swings in blood glucose readings. Nerve damage in the abdomen can also produce intermittent diarrhoea or incomplete bladder emptying, which can lead to persistent infections of the bladder and kidneys. Abdominal nerve damage may also produce faintness or dizziness when standing up from a chair or getting out of bed.

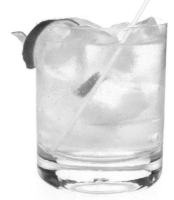

Keep good glucose control to prevent nerve damage

The best way to treat or control nerve damage is to maintain good control of your diabetes through the relevant parts of the critical five-point plan: diet, exercise and medical supervision.

Nerve damage is most commonly felt and most easily detected in the feet. Your doctor or podiatrist can easily test nerve response with tiny needles and by testing the reflexes in the knee and ankle.

It is vital that diabetics have a foot inspection regularly, perhaps every six months. Any sores or ulcers or severe tingling sensations should be reported immediately.

Diabetics should also tell their doctor about any digestive complaints and avoid excessive consumption of alcohol, which also acts on the nerves.

Some nerve problems in the wrist can be fixed with a simple operation.

Infections of the bladder, kidneys and vagina

Diabetics have a higher rate of infections of the vagina, bladder and kidney. Their urine, semen and secretions of the vagina have higher levels of glucose, which provides a better environment for growth of germs or fungi.

Infections of the bladder (cystitis) and kidney (pyelonephritis) are more common in women because of the short length of the urethra, the tube that takes urine out of the body. Germs can travel up this tube during sexual intercourse so it is always wise to empty the bladder after intercourse to flush out the germs.

Nerve damage in the bladder may cause incomplete emptying of the bladder, which helps promote growth of germs.

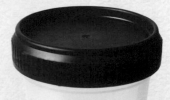

Use your five-point plan to prevent infections

Once again, the best way to prevent and control infections is to manage your glucose levels through the relevant parts of the five-point plan: diet, exercise and medical supervision.

Prompt treatment can prevent chronic kidney damage or kidney failure. Symptoms of bladder and kidney infections are passing small amounts of urine at more frequent intervals and a burning feeling or pain when passing urine. Sometimes backache is associated with a kidney infection. Report any symptoms you experience to your doctor immediately.

Bladder and kidney infections can be diagnosed with urine tests and are usually cleared up with antibiotics.

Symptoms of infections of the vagina or penis are itching and discharges. These infections can be treated with ointments or pessaries.

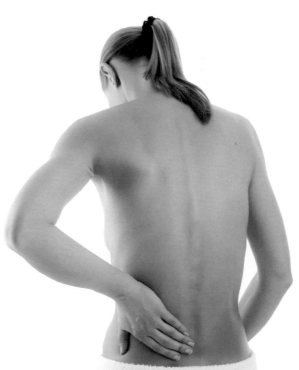

Erectile dysfunction and diabetes

Australian studies indicate that between 50 and 60 per cent of diabetic men over the age of 50 suffer erectile dysfunction. In the US, there are more than 25 million men with erectile dysfunction – and they are not all diabetics.

Erectile dysfunction (ED), or impotence, occurs when the penis no longer becomes fully erect, remains erect or becomes erect at all.

Until the 1970s, doctors thought most impotence was caused by psychological factors. Now they believe about 70 per cent is caused by physical factors and 30 per cent by psychological reasons.

Blood vessel damage and nerve damage associated with diabetes are common causes. But ED can also be caused by depression, stress, anxiety, relationship difficulties, heavy smoking or drinking.

Diabetics can have an active and normal sex life

There is no reason why diabetics cannot have a normal and active sex life. As men get older, they are more likely to experience erectile dysfunction – regardless of whether they have diabetes.

In diabetics, impotence may occur slowly over many years or it may happen suddenly. Either way, there are effective treatments available. It is common among diabetic men to experience a drop in sexual desire because of high blood glucose levels. So the first rule is to follow your general diabetic management plan to maintain healthy blood glucose levels.

Doctors may order a few blood tests or place an injection into the shaft of the penis to confirm what is causing the problem. If a doctor believes the ED is caused by psychological problems, the preferred treatment may be sexual counselling and education, usually with the partner.

For physical causes, a doctor may discuss a penile implant, either in the form of a malleable rod or an inflatable device. Another popular method is injections done by the patient or his partner to open up the blood vessels. Patients may also try a vacuum-type device to create blood flow, which is then trapped with a rubber band around the base of the penis.

Most recently, millions of men have used sildenafil (Viagra or similar drugs), which blocks an enzyme in the penis that breaks down a chemical produced during sexual stimulation. The chemical helps produce an erection. These drugs have been found to be effective in about 60 per cent of diabetic men with ED. However, they can have side effects such as headache, flushing, stuffy nose and diarrhoea. And they should not be taken with nitroglycerin (an anti-angina drug) because they interact and cause low blood pressure.

Diabetes hits immune system, teeth and other parts

Diabetes can slow the action of white blood cells, an important part of the immune system. This can inhibit your ability to fight infections.

Diabetics are three times more likely to die of complications from influenza or pneumonia, according to the US Center for Disease Control in Atlanta.

There is also evidence that diabetes produces lower thyroid levels (hypothyroidism), especially in women over 40.

Diabetics have an increased risk of tooth decay and gum disease because high blood glucose levels can reduce the flow of saliva and inhibit infection-fighting white blood cells.

Diabetics can also develop red or yellowish spots around the elbows or knees (xanthoma and xanthelasma) if they have excessive fat in the blood or poor glucose control.

There can also be swelling of the ankles and face, skin sores on the shins or skin problems at the suite of insulin injections.

Indeed, there are few parts of the body that are not affected by diabetes.

Good control – the key to all the problems

Good management of your diabetes is the key to any of the complications of the disease.

Diabetics should be especially careful about dental hygiene, brushing at least twice a day with a soft brush and having their teeth and gums checked regularly by a dentist.

Diabetics should talk to their doctor about having an annual flu injection. Older diabetics should also discuss a pneumonia injection.

If you notice anything unusual happening to your body, it should be reported to your doctor because it could be diabetes-related. The earlier the complications are detected, the sooner they can be treated effectively before they cause major problems.

And if that was not depressing enough ...

People with diabetes are more likely to suffer depression. It is not clear how the link works but it is there.

A review of studies found that depression was associated with a 60 per cent increase of type 2 diabetes while type 2 diabetes was only associated with a 15 per cent increase in risk of depression.

Other studies cited by the International Diabetes Federation show a higher rate of complications amongst diabetics with depression. And diabetics with depression are generally much less capable of controlling their diabetes.

Finally, the studies have shown that diabetics with depression have a significantly higher risk of death compared with patients who have only one of the conditions.

The health costs of diabetics with depression are 4.5 times those of diabetics without depression, according to an American study (Daniel Chapman et al, The Vital Link between Chronic Diseases and Depressive Disorders, 2005).

One of the problems with early recognition and treatment of depression is the difficulty in separating the symptoms of depression from the symptoms of poor diabetes control.

Watch for symptoms of depression and act

It is not surprising that people with diabetes become anxious or depressed about developing long-term complications of diabetes. Reading only the left-hand pages of this book would be enough!

Diabetics should not be ashamed of feeling gloomy sometimes. And they should certainly take encouragement from the right-hand pages in this book!

The important thing is to recognise the symptoms and get some help. Diabetics need to stay positive and motivated to fight their disease. As this book has tried to show, it is a fight that can be won but it requires constant vigilance and enthusiasm as well as a sense of challenge and fun. Depression can subdue these motivating forces, so the depression has to be recognised and addressed.

These are some of the symptoms:

- Feeling anxious or tearful, or losing appetite
- Regularly feeling sad, pessimistic or hopeless or feeling unable to enjoy activities
- Lack of interest in your usual relationships and activities
- Difficulty in sleeping or waking up very early in the morning
- Feeling constantly lethargic and short of energy

If you are feeling one or more of these symptoms and are having trouble controlling your diabetes, go to your doctor who may arrange counselling or antidepressant tablets or both.

Top 10 nations for incidence of diabetes

Country/Territory	Millions of cases	National Prevalence %
1. China	98.4	9.62
2. India	65.1	8.56
3. USA	24.4	10.9
4. Brazil	11.9	9.0
5. Russian Federation	10.9	10.03
6. Mexico	8.7	11.8
7. Indonesia	8.6	5.6
8. Germany	7.6	11.9
9. Egypt	7.5	15.56
10. Japan	7.2	7.6

Source: International Diabetes Federation Diabetes Atlas, Sixth Edition, 2013 Update. Figures are adult cases

The diabetes diet is great for general health

The diet that is best for diabetics is also a great diet for your heart and all-round health.

Like most things about managing diabetes, the eating rules are simple and should quickly become second nature. The overall goal is to stop putting junk in your mouth.

Here are the five main principles:

1. Get most of your kilojoules from carbohydrates – especially those that are not refined and those that are rich in vitamins and minerals. Good examples are wholegrain breads, pasta, rice (Basmati or Doongarra), legumes and fruit.
2. Choose protein foods in moderation. Stick to lean meat, skinless chicken, fish, eggs, soy beans and tofu.
3. Choose food high in fibre – wholegrain breads, fruits and vegetables.
4. Avoid saturated fats as much as possible – butter, cream, cheese, processed snacks and many fried take-away foods.
5. Avoid foods and beverages very high in sugar and low in other nutrients – sweets and lollies, sugary soft drinks and cordials.

Let us examine each of these five principles in a little more detail.

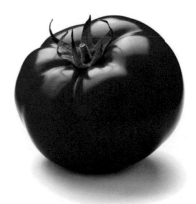

Choose mainly carbohydrates

Carbohydrates should make up more than half the calories/kilojoules in your eating plan. Experts say that means 230-315g of carbohydrates per day for women and 350-474g for men. Aim to have at least two serves of carbohydrate-based foods at each meal and eat mainly carbohydrates for snacks.

Carbohydrates provide the body with energy. When carbohydrates are digested, they are converted to glucose, which enters the blood stream as energy. This is why it is important to have a steady intake of carbohydrates during the day. This is even more important for diabetics on medication and insulin.

The major sources of carbohydrates should be wholegrain breads and cereals, pasta, Basmati or Doongara rice, fruits and legumes such as beans and lentils. Sugar is a type of carbohydrate and can be eaten in moderation by diabetics, especially if it is part of a healthy diet and your food plan is otherwise good. But avoid foods that are high in sugar and calories or are totally comprised of sugar or sugar and fat.

Some dry biscuits are high in carbohydrates, particularly those with grains. Examples of good legume choice include beaked beans (check labels for those brands lower in salt), kidney beans, chick peas and three and four-bean mixes. Good starchy vegetables including potatoes, sweet potatoes, yams and sweet corn are good choices. Other vegetables may be lower in carbohydrates but should be eaten for other reasons including for their vitamins and minerals.

Choose protein foods in moderation

Our bodies need protein for growth and repair of tissues. Try to make protein up to a fifth of each meal. Proteins are also a source of energy. But many protein foods such as meat contain high levels of fat, sometimes hidden. Excessive protein can damage your kidneys.

Choose lean meat. It is far more nutritious than products such as sausages, pies and processed meats, which are higher in unhealthy saturated fats and often loaded with salt.

Fish is an excellent source of protein and contains healthy fats such as omega-3 oil, which can protect against heart disease, an ever-present risk for diabetics. Canned salmon and tuna are a superb source of protein and good oil as well as calcium. Canned fish is also a great snack option but be careful of some of the fancy sauces now sold in small cans of fish; some are too fatty and salty. Fish in spring water or tomato is usually safer, possibly with added herbs, lemon and pepper.

Poultry is a better option than red meat. Strike the skin off the chicken or turkey; you can almost halve the calories in a piece of chicken by talking off the skin. Make sure you avoid cooking meat and poultry in saturated fats – use olive oil, low-fat margarine or vegetable oil but not palm or coconut oils.

Eggs, not fried, are a good source of protein but should be limited to less than one a day because of their fat content. With other dairy products, choose low-fat options. Tofu is an excellent source of protein, but not a favourite of mine unless spiced up.

Nuts are a good protein source, but are also fatty so eat in moderation. Seeds such as sunflower, pumpkin, linseed and sesame are rich in omega-3 oils and other goodness.

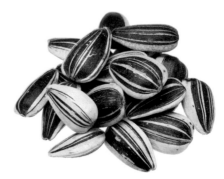

Choose foods high in fibre

High fibre foods tend to be low in fat and kilojoules. Vegetables, fruit and legumes provide some energy but are also packed with vitamins, minerals and fibre. They also tend to make you feel full. Experts say you should consume about 30g of fibre a day, easily achieved in a sensible diet that includes fruit, vegetables, cereals and grains.

There are two types of fibre – soluble and insoluble. Soluble fibre can be found in oats, legumes, barley, fruit and vegetables. It may help lower cholesterol. Insoluble fibre is found in grain and grain products such as bread, pasta and cereal, especially wholegrain varieties. This type of fibre can prevent constipation and other bowel problems.

Try to eat at least five serves of vegetables and two serves of fruit each day.

One of the main roles of fibre is to keep your digestive system healthy. A high fibre diet is even more important for older people because the digestive system slows down with age. Disorders that can arise from a low fibre diet include constipation, haemorrhoids, irritable bowel syndrome, diverticulitis, heart disease and some cancers.

An example of a daily diet with more than 35g of fibre would include 2 cereal biscuits, 4 slices of wholegrain bread, 1 tablespoon of peanut butter, 2 pieces of fruit, 1 cup of frozen vegetables, 1 small boiled potato with skin, 1 cup of pasta, 2 wholemeal dry biscuits, 25 almonds and 1 cup of fresh fruit juice.

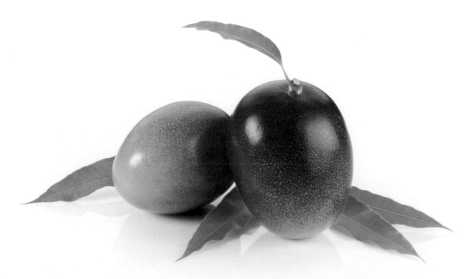

Avoid saturated fats

This is the big one for diabetics as well as people fighting heart disease or weight problems. There is no guidance more important than avoiding saturated fats. They have more kilojoules than any other food, make diabetes control more difficult and damage your heart by raising cholesterol.

Many foods have visible fat; you can see it clearly in the meat or the skin on poultry and in butter, margarine, oils, lard and cream. Other foods have fats that are more difficult to see or are invisible. These include processed meats, cakes, pastries, biscuits, many take-away foods, snack foods, potato chips, gravies and sauces.

Many nutritionists say fat should provide no more than 20-30% of your daily energy intake, with saturated fat providing no more than 7%. The recommended daily intake of all fat is 25 to 40g for an average person trying to lose weight. Active people can consume a little more.

There are three main types of fat in food and all have different effects on blood cholesterol.

Saturated fats are the ones that raised your blood cholesterol. Found in fatty meats, full-fat dairy products, many beaked products and two vegetable oils – coconut and palm oil.

Polyunsaturated fats are healthier and can help lower blood cholesterol if your meals are low in saturated fats. Found in many vegetable oils, fish, soybean, nuts and seeds. Omega-3 is one of these fats.

Monounsaturated fats can also help lower blood cholesterol if your diet is low in saturated fats. Found in some spreads containing olive oil and canola. Eat in moderation because they are high in kilojoules.

Australia

Adult population (aged 20–79)	16.5 million
Prevalence of adult diabetes	10.0%
Total numbers	1.65 million
Diabetes deaths	9,765 per year

Source: IDF Diabetes Atlas, Sixth Edition, 2013.

Canada

Adult population (aged 20–79)	25.8 million
Prevalence of adult diabetes	10.21%
Total numbers	2.6 million
Diabetes deaths	17,239

Source: IDF Diabetes Atlas, Sixth Edition, 2013.

China

Adult population (aged 20–79)	123 million
Prevalence of adult diabetes	9.62%
Total numbers	98.4 million
Diabetes deaths	1.3 million

Source: IDF Diabetes Atlas, Sixth Edition, 2013.

France

Adult population (aged 20–79)	45 million
Prevalence of adult diabetes	7.5%
Total numbers	3.4 million
Diabetes deaths	22,953

Source: IDF Diabetes Atlas, Sixth Edition, 2013.

Avoid foods high in sugar and low in other nutrients

Some sugar can be included in a healthy eating plan. It is no longer the number one villain in diabetes control. Sugar that is contained in otherwise nutritional food such as fruit, yoghurt and some breakfast cereals does not need to be avoided – just watch the kilojoules and fat.

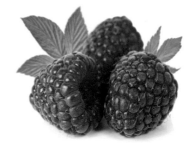

A teaspoon of sugar on your porridge or cereal may not necessarily upset your diabetes control. Honey is also a good option. Eating a little sugar this way does not raise your blood glucose as much as eating sugar on its own or in sweets, biscuits, sugary drinks and other sugar products.

The main problem with sugar for diabetics is that it puts on weight. There is still a place for artificial sweeteners, particularly aspartame and Stevia, which continue to get favourable reviews in the scientific media.

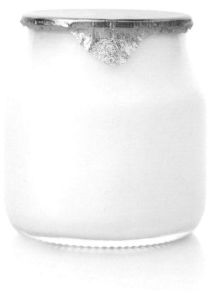

Realistic goals will lead to real rewards

The food plan for diabetics must become a way of life, not a temporary diet.

Most people who go on a crash diet or fad diet end up weighing more than when they started.

Resist the urge to set unattainable weight loss goals based on television world records. It is better to lose a kilogram or a couple of pounds a month for 12 months than lose 12 kilograms or 25 pounds in a month only to put it back on later.

Cut yourself a bit of slack. I aim to get 19 meals out of 21 just about perfectly in line with the eating principles, allowing two meals a week for special occasions, dining out or as a reward. Those two meals are not a licence to lash out, but a margin for error which might mean a piece of cheese or a slightly wicked dessert if my blood glucose levels are under control.

Alcohol is not banned in a diabetic diet, but it should be restricted to a maximum of one or two drinks a day. And remember most alcoholic drinks deliver dead calories and some load you up with sugar. If you take alcohol, be prepared to be tougher on yourself with food intake and exercise. My preference was to avoid alcohol and give myself some slack on food.

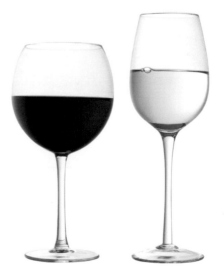

It all starts with breakfast

In many ways, breakfast is the easiest meal to get right. It's an important meal because it kick-starts your metabolism after a prolonged fasting period.

Eating a substantial breakfast can make you feel less hungry during the day and it becomes easier to avoid junky snacks.

Start with a piece of fresh fruit or its juice, not the sugar-laden drinks labelled juice drinks in many supermarkets.

For a cereal, use oats in the most unprocessed form you can find. For variety, substitute with one of the wheat biscuit products available in supermarkets, preferably the one with least salt. Use no-fat or low-fat milk. Avoid sugar; if necessary use a sugar substitute containing aspartame or stevia (the two sugar substitute products which seem to get the best reviews from dieticians and doctors).

Eat one or two slices of wholegrain bread or toast. Use margarine or a spread with less than 40 per cent total fat, less than 10 per cent saturated fat and less than 400mg per gram of salt. Spreads containing plant sterols will lower cholesterol absorption, but they are significantly more expensive. Jams can vary in sugar content from 20 per cent to 80 per cent; choose low. An egg a day is also acceptable.

Hot tea or coffee is fine, but try to avoid sugar and fatty milk. And water is a great way to finish a meal.

Germany

Adult population (aged 20–79)	63 million
Prevalence of adult diabetes	11.95%
Total numbers	7.6 million
Diabetes deaths	62,460

Source: IDF Diabetes Atlas, Sixth Edition, 2013.

Greece

Adult population (aged 20–79)	8.3 million
Prevalence of adult diabetes	7.0%
Total numbers	585,000
Diabetes deaths	4,906

Source: IDF Diabetes Atlas, Sixth Edition, 2013.

India

Adult population (aged 20–79)	760 million
Prevalence of adult diabetes	8.56%
Total numbers	65 million
Diabetes deaths	1,065,053

Source: IDF Diabetes Atlas, Sixth Edition, 2013.

Indonesia

Adult population (aged 20–79)	154 million
Prevalence of adult diabetes	5.5%
Total numbers	8.6 million
Diabetes deaths	172,600

Source: IDF Diabetes Atlas, Sixth Edition, 2013.

Take up the challenge to food makers

The food and beverage industry is one of the biggest industries in the world. It spends billions of dollars marketing their products, trying to persuade consumers to buy more. This should be no surprise because the main function of food manufacturing companies is to make a profit.

It is also no surprise that these companies should try to make their products taste as good as possible so people buy more food more frequently.

Therefore they target our strongest and most sensitive taste buds – sugar, fat and salt. These are the three ingredients most damaging to our health if taken in excess.

Diabetics should eat as little packaged and processed food as possible. They should read food labels carefully. It is best to avoid any processed foods containing more than 400mg per gram of salt. Try to avoid processed foods containing more than 10 per cent fat (except margarine, cooking oils or other products used in in very small quantities), especially if most of the fat is saturated or trans fat. The lower the sugar content the better, but a maximum of 10 per cent is a good guide unless in a product used in very small quantities such as a jam.

The good news is that food manufacturers are beginning to get the message about consumer demand for healthier food and there are many more healthier choices available in supermarkets. The not-so-good news is that sometimes a no-sugar food can be laden with fat, or vice versa. Some fat-free products have far too much sugar. This is all aimed at connecting with one of your three magic taste bud buttons. Be smart enough to beat their tricks.

Learn some of the tricks of the supermarket foods

'**Cholesterol-free**' labels can be misleading because it does not necessarily mean the product is low in fat. It is the saturated fat in food that raises the cholesterol in our blood rather than cholesterol from food. Vegetable oils often use the 'cholesterol-free' label, which might be true but cholesterol is only found in animal products anyway. Some vegetable oils such as palm oil and coconut oil can be high in saturated fats. Look for oils or margarines that are free of trans fats and less than 10 per cent saturated fat. It is possible to find some margarines with less than 30 per cent fat.

'**Lite**'/ '**Light**' does not necessarily mean the food is low in calories/kilojoules. It may refer to texture, colour or flavour.

'**Reduced Fat**' / '**Reduced Salt**' These terms mean that the product has less fat or salt than the regular version. It does not necessarily mean it is low in fat or salt. Reduced fat cheese labelled 25 per cent less than the original version can still be high in fat if the original version is very high. Check the label.

'**94% Fat-Free**' sounds great and it is in some products. But it is above the legal threshold that would allow it to be labelled 'Low Fat' or 'Low in Fat'. There are many milks, yoghurts or other products with much lower fat content.

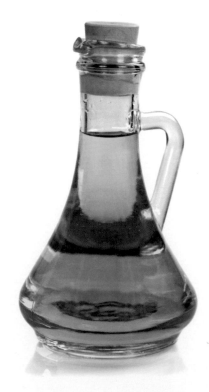

A word about GI

The Glycaemic Index (GI) is a relatively new concept which helps diabetics choose their food to help control their blood glucose.

GI is a ranking system for the length of time it takes for carbohydrates in foods to make your blood glucose levels rise. Some carbohydrates make your glucose levels rise quickly and are called high GI foods. Others make your blood glucose levels rise slowly and are called low GI foods.

Low GI foods are your best choice, but you do not need to eliminate high GI foods. The trick is to mix high with low, to balance a high GI food with a low GI food in the same meal. Doctors say that having at least one low GI food in each meal will not only lower your blood glucose levels, but will also increase the effectiveness of insulin, reduce hunger and lower cholesterol.

Foods with a low GI include legumes such as lentils and beans, pasta, most orchard fruit, wholegrain bread, yoghurt and traditional porridge.

Carbohydrates with a high GI include most rice, most potatoes, biscuits and some refined cereals.

It is not wise to choose foods on GI alone. Some foods with a moderate GI have a high fat content. Use GI as a second-order check on your food plan after you have applied the five principles of good eating and kept your total calorie/kilojoule intake to an appropriate level.

Italy

Adult population (aged 20–79)	45.6 million
Prevalence of adult diabetes	7.95%
Total numbers	3.6 million
Diabetes deaths	26,728

Source: IDF Diabetes Atlas, Sixth Edition, 2013.

Japan

Adult population (aged 20–79)	95 million
Prevalence of adult diabetes	7.56%
Total numbers	7.2 million
Diabetes deaths	64,680

Source: IDF Diabetes Atlas, Sixth Edition, 2013.

New Zealand

Adult population (aged 20–79)	3.1 million
Prevalence of adult diabetes	10.97%
Total numbers	343,000
Diabetes deaths	2,145

Source: IDF Diabetes Atlas, Sixth Edition, 2013.

Russia

Adult population (aged 20–79)	109 million
Prevalence of adult diabetes	10.03%
Total numbers	10.9 million
Diabetes deaths	197,300

Source: IDF Diabetes Atlas, Sixth Edition, 2013.

How common foods rate for GI

Foods with low GI: Apples, bananas, oranges, sweet potatoes, lentils, chick peas, kidney beans, green peas, baked beans, traditional porridge, rolled oats, multigrain bread, peanuts, low-fat yoghurt, low-fat milk, milk chocolate

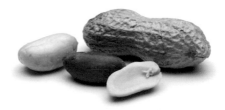

Foods with medium GI: Melons, pineapples, new potatoes, beetroot, Basmati rice, instant porridge, wholemeal bread, rye bread, muesli bars, full-fat ice cream, cranberry juice, digestive biscuits

Foods with high GI: Parsnips, broad beans, mashed potatoes, boiled potatoes, baked potatoes, instant rice, white rice, cornflakes, puffed rice, bagels, white bread, brown bread, doughnuts, tapioca, glucose drink, rice cake

The GI ranking system uses a scale from 1 to 100, with 70 or more being a high GI and scores of 55 or below considered low GI. Remember that GI is not necessarily the prime consideration in your food choice. Some food manufacturers are exploiting the popularity of GI ratings by promoting low GI foods which are high in fat or sugar. It is more important to consider the GI in the context of a whole meal rather than one ingredient.

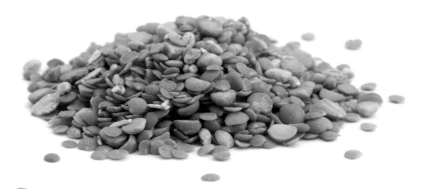

Top 10 tips for a flying start to your eating plan

1. Eat smaller portions. Limit meat, chicken and fish serving sizes to the palm of your hand – 200g instead of 500g.
2. Switch to no-fat milk or 1% fat milk. By doing this, if you consumer an average of half a litre of milk per day, you are saving 126g of fat per week, compared to full cream milk.
3. Choose a good margarine product and stick to it. Look for spread that is less than 40% fat and less than 10% saturated fat.
4. Select a low-fat (less than 5 per cent) yoghurt and keep a good stock for snacks, desserts and breakfast. Yoghurt is a versatile source of calcium and protein as well as adding some sweetness. Use plain yoghurt on vegetables to add moisture.
5. Steal the best eating habits from other cultures to create a healthy multicultural diet. Eat French by eating small portions and taking small mouthfuls before chewing slowly. Eat Japanese by putting more fish in your diet. East Asian by including lots of rice and vegetables. Americans? Yes, even the Americans have one good eating habit – water on the table and salad before main course. But don't spoil the salad benefit by adding fat-filled dressings.
6. Learn about spices. Pepper, curry, chilli and other spices can add taste to a healthy diet that might otherwise seem bland in the absence of large amounts of fat, sugar and salt.
7. Try the range of Weight Watchers to find any that suit your palate. Some won't, but it's a bonus if you find one or two that work for you.
8. If you MUST have cheese occasionally, use small pieces of strongly-flavoured cheese to satisfy your craving.
9. An apple a day can keep the doctor away. And the cardiologist. And the endocrinologist. Apples have good carbohydrates, vitamins, minerals and water and are converted to glucose relatively slowly. They are a great snack or dessert.
10. Salsa is a good snack or garnish. Dice fresh tomatoes, onions and chilli peppers and add pepper, garlic and other spices to suit your taste.

Top 10 tips for reducing fat intake

1. Grill, dry roast or steam meat rather than fry.

2. Use lean meats such as veal or skinless chicken breasts.

3. Eat fish more often.

4. Steam, boil or stir-fry vegetables (use minimum oil, preferably olive oil).

5. Select low-fat biscuits.

6. Use 'no-fat' salad dressings.

7. Use skim milk or no-fat milk and fat-reduced dairy products, preferably containing less than 10% fat.

8. Top vegetables and meat with low-fat cheeses, yoghurt or vegetable sauces for taste.

9. Prepare meat sauces, casseroles and soups ahead of time; refrigerate and remove fat before adding vegetables or thickening.

10. Learn how to use dozens of spices to add flavour to food while reducing the tasty fat, salt and sugar in your eating plan.

Saudi Arabia

Adult population (aged 20–79)	18.1 million
Prevalence of adult diabetes	20.2%
Total numbers	3.7 million
Diabetes deaths	22,113

Source: IDF Diabetes Atlas, Sixth Edition, 2013.

United Arab Emirates

Adult population (aged 20–79)	7.4 million
Prevalence of adult diabetes	10.02%
Total numbers	764,000
Diabetes deaths	1,385

Source: IDF Diabetes Atlas, Sixth Edition, 2013.

United Kingdom

Adult population (aged 20–79)	45.3 million
Prevalence of adult diabetes	6.57%
Total numbers	3 million
Diabetes deaths	24,897

Source: IDF Diabetes Atlas, Sixth Edition, 2013.

United States

Adult population (aged 20–79)	224 million
Prevalence of adult diabetes	10.9%
Total numbers	24.4 million
Diabetes deaths	192,725

Source: IDF Diabetes Atlas, Sixth Edition, 2013.

Top 10 tips for eating out

1. Drink some water and eat a piece of fruit before going to the restaurant, it will make you less hungry.

2. Ask for wholegrain bread and avoid the butter.

3. Foods described as sautéed, fried, crispy, pan-fried, creamed, basted, au lait and butter-sauced are likely to be high in fat.

4. Consider a second starter for your main meal, perhaps with a salad on the side.

5. Pasta is a good option. Consider starter size and choose vegetable or vegetable-based sauces rather than cream or cheese sauces.

6. Baked or boiled potatoes without butter are better than roast, sautéed or mashed potatoes.

7. Don't hesitate to ask about cooking methods, including type of fat used, or ask for skin to be removed from poultry or for a small portion of meat.

8. Ask for sauces – including salad dressings – to be served on the side so you can control your intake. Do not hesitate to leave some food uneaten if your hunger is satisfied.

9. Finish with fresh fruit or a fruit-based dessert. Maybe share with a friend to reduce calories.

10. Drink water rather than sugary drinks. Use diet mixers if drinking alcoholic spirits.

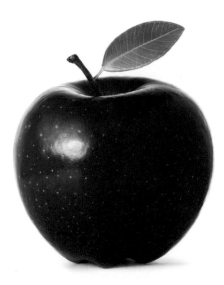

Top 10 tips for calorie-crunching some common foods

1. Cut the calories in your pizza base by 50% by choosing a thin crust.

2. Cut the croutons and dressing from Caesar salad and reduce the calories by almost 50% as well as reducing the fat. Use a low-calorie no-fat dressing instead.

3. Choose a can of minestrone or vegetable soup instead of cream of tomato and cut the calories by more than half. Better still, make your own vegetable soup.

4. Drink a regular black espresso coffee rather than a cappuccino or latte and say goodbye to more than 250 kilojoules. Drink diet soft drinks and save more than 500 kilojoules per can.

5. Remove the skin from chicken breasts and save half the kilojoules.

6. Swap a medium bacon, lettuce and tomato sandwich for a medium salmon and cucumber sandwich and save 1000 kilojoules.

7. Use 100g of tomato sauce instead of carbonara sauce on pasta and save 500 kilojoules.

8. Grill, steam, bake or microwave your meats and fish rather than frying. Place meat on a rack in the oven to drain excess fat.

9. Use 50g of cottage cheese instead of cheddar and save nearly 700 kilojoules.

10. Low-fat yoghurt is a terrific option for breakfast, snacks, soups, salads and desserts.

Top 10 tips for take-away

1. Make your healthy choices before visiting a take-away outlet. Visit the websites of the big take-away chains to study the nutritional contents of their products. There are surprising differences in different products.

2. Choose water or diet versions of soft drinks.

3. Avoid the sauces offered for salads and other foods; they can sometimes double the calories.

4. Order wholegrain bread or rolls, non-dairy spreads and good protein fillings with salad.

5. Do not be fooled by 'cholesterol-free' or 'vegetable oils only' signs in fried food shops. Palm oil and coconut oil are just as bad as animal fat.

6. Noodles are a good choice but choose an accompaniment low in fat – vegetables, fish or lean meat.

7. Avoid pies, hot dogs, pastries and fries.

8. Japanese food is a wonderful choice, especially sushi, sashimi and rice rolls with vegetables or fish.

9. Stir-fry vegetables with tofu, lean meat or fish is a sound choice.

10. Choose boiled rice rather than fried rice.

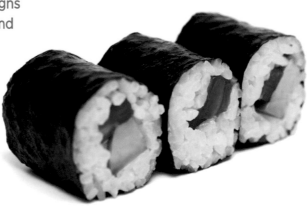

Recipes
Breakfast

Roasted Plums & Ricotta on Rye

This dish is great to have for breakfast, lunch or as a snack. Divided between two, it's a generous serving of 2 plums each but this can be cut back for individual tastes or needs. Dark rye is a better choice than white bread or even some wholegrain varieties, but is still to be consumed in moderation. It has a low glycemic index, has a higher fibre content than other breads and also boasts a good level of magnesium.

Serves 2

4 small plums (any variety)
Dash of extra virgin olive oil
½ tsp vanilla powder
1 tsp cinnamon
½ cup (130g) smooth ricotta
2 slices dark rye bread
Micro greens or watercress for serving (optional)

1. Preheat the oven to 180°C/356°F.
2. Halve plums, remove stones and place in a shallow baking dish. Sprinkle over the olive oil, vanilla powder and cinnamon and bake for 20 minutes until tender.
3. Spread each slice of bread with ricotta and top with roasted plums and micro greens or watercress.

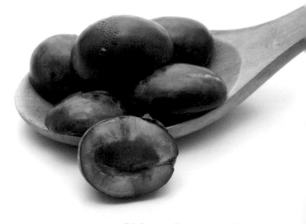

Bacon Cups with Turmeric Eggs

These bacon cups are handy to make and have ready to go in the refrigerator or enjoy fresh out of the oven. You can add vegetables to the cups or play around with spices and flavour combinations. Turmeric is a powerhouse spice and sits on the must-use list for diabetics. It's a strong antioxidant and anti-inflammatory that helps regulate insulin, balance blood glucose and help prevent insulin resistance. A word of caution if you have never cooked with turmeric before, it has a potent yellow colour that will stain anything that comes into contact with it, such as bench tops, utensils, skin or clothing. Be careful when using and if a spill occurs clean it up immediately.

Serves 2

4 rashers bacon
4 eggs
2 spring onions (scallions), chopped
1 tsp turmeric powder
Sea salt and black pepper

1. Preheat the oven to 180°C/356°F.
2. Lightly grease 4 holes in a muffin tin with olive oil and lay one bacon rasher in each hole.
3. Cook bacon for 5 minutes to begin crisping it up.
4. Remove tray from the oven and crack one egg into each hole. Sprinkle over chopped spring onions, turmeric, salt and pepper and return to the oven to bake for a further 10 minutes or until the egg is cooked to your liking.

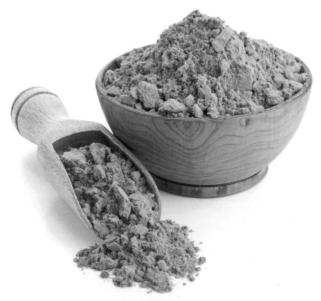

Mediterranean Breakfast Plate

Delicious breakfast ideas don't come easier than this. Taking inspiration from the Mediterranean, where longevity and happiness are directly attributed to lifestyle and diet, this breakfast plate can be eaten at any time of the day.

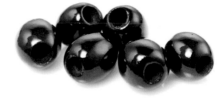

Serves 1

1 egg
Pinch of sea salt
½ tsp ground cumin
½ cup (125g) hummus
1 small Lebanese cucumber, diced
½ tomato, diced
¼ cup (40g) black olives
1 cup (50g) shredded lettuce, any variety
¼ cup (25g) Greek feta cheese, crumbled (optional)

1. Whisk the eggs with sea salt and cumin.
2. Heat a small frying pan and scramble the egg, set aside.
3. Use a good quality store-bought hummus or prepare your own by adding 1 cup (200g) of cooked chickpeas to the bowl of a food processor with 1 tbsp hulled tahini, the juice of half a lemon, ¼ cup (60ml) extra virgin olive oil and salt and pepper to taste. Mix until smooth in texture.
4. Place all components on a place and drizzle a small amount of extra virgin olive oil over the top.

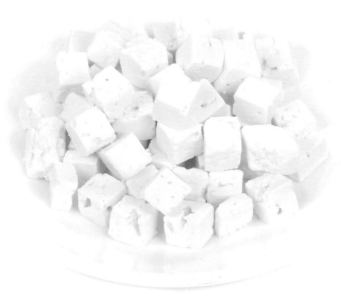

Sprouted Lentil Salad with Fried Eggs

Sprout your own lentils

You can use quality store bought lentils and bean sprouts or try at sprouting your own at home.

2 cups of dried lentils or beans of choice
Glass jar
Muslin or breathable cloth to cover the jar

1. Soak lentils or beans in filtered water overnight or for up to 14 hours.
2. Rinse thoroughly and drain any excess liquid.
3. Place lentils in the jar and cover the top with the cloth, secure with a rubber band.
4. Store the jar on a kitchen counter and rinse the lentils once a day, making sure to drain any water before returning the lentils to the jar.
5. The lentils or beans should begin sprouting after 3 days. Test one before rinsing the lentils one final time. Return sprouted lentils to the jar and secure the cloth on the top. Store in the refrigerator and eat within two weeks. If the lentils are slimy or smell off-putting bin the batch and begin again.

Serves 1

1 cup (200g) sprouted lentils or beans (e.g. mung beans)
½ cup (100g) artichoke hearts (store-bought in brine
is fine)
1-inch piece of fresh ginger, grated
Juice and zest of ½ lemon
Pinch of sea salt and black pepper
1 – 2 eggs

1. In a small bowl combine lentils, artichokes, fresh ginger, lemon juice and zest. Stir, taste and adjust seasoning with sea salt and black pepper.
2. In a small frying pan, cook eggs to your liking, sunny side up or over easy.
3. Serve the fried eggs on top of the lentil salad.

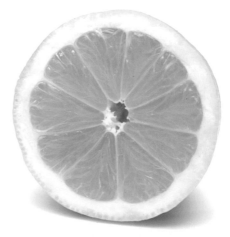

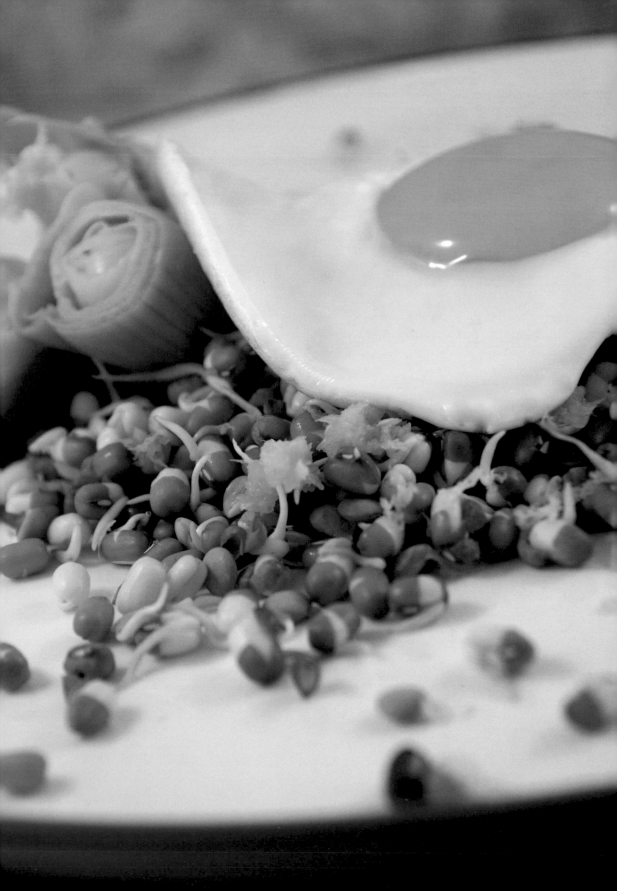

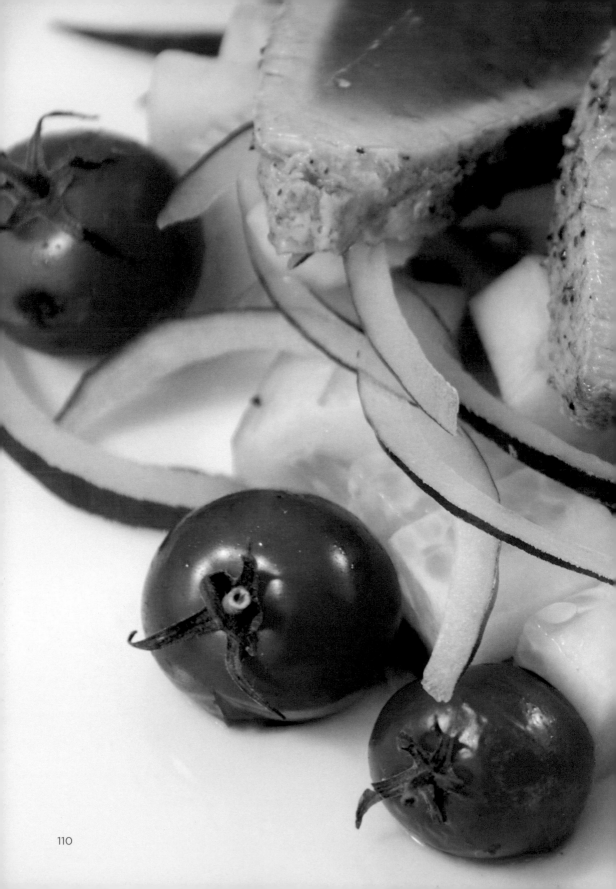

Salads

Simple tuna salad

When we think of a tuna salad, most of us envisage a tin of tuna that we empty onto a plate with a few leaves and seasonings. It's not hard to cook a tuna steak at home if you have access to good quality fresh tuna, and it makes the world of difference in texture and taste. Keep the salad simple with additional seasonings so you can really appreciate the natural flavour of the fish.

Serves 1

8 cherry tomatoes
1 small cucumber
¼ Spanish (red) onion (optional)
150g – 180g (5-6oz) fresh tuna steak
Sea salt & black pepper
Extra virgin olive oil

1. In a pan, drizzle a small amount of extra virgin olive oil and cook the cherry tomatoes for 3 – 4 minutes until the skin begins to darken and the tomatoes soften. Set aside.
2. Dice cucumber and finely slice red onion if using.
3. Season both sides of the tuna steak with sea salt and black pepper; use your hands to press the seasoning into the flesh.
4. Heat a small pan with a drizzle of extra virgin olive oil. Lay the tuna steak into the hot pan and cook 1 – 2 minutes a side. Set aside to rest for 4 minutes.
5. Slice the tuna steak and assemble the salad by laying the tuna on top of the cucumber, red onion and tomatoes. Drizzle a small amount of extra virgin olive oil over the top if desired.

Pumpkin & Prosciutto Salad

This is a great flavour combination with sweet and spicy pumpkin mixed with salty prosciutto. While you may not serve this salad on its own, it makes a great accompaniment to a roasted chicken or beef fillet, or served alongside falafel for a vegetarian option.

Serves 2

250g (8.8oz) butternut (or other variety) pumpkin
3 tbsp coconut oil, melted
1 tbsp chilli flakes
2 tsp smoked paprika
2 cups (134g) baby kale
150-180g (5-6oz) thinly sliced prosciutto or pancetta

1. Preheat the oven to 180°C/350°F and line an oven tray with baking paper.
2. Slice the pumpkin into chunks or crescents of an even thickness. Lay on the baking tray and pour over the coconut oil, chilli flakes and paprika. Roast in the oven for 20 – 30 minutes or until soft and slightly caramelised on top.
3. On a platter spread out the baby kale and half the prosciutto.
4. Place the roasted pumpkin on top and then scatter the remaining prosciutto around the pumpkin.

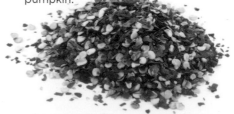

Soba noodle salad with prawns and chilli lime dressing

Soba noodles are a great alternative to pasta. Along with rice noodles, good quality soba noodles make a great salad with prawns and a spicy dressing, and it can be on the table in less than 10 minutes if you have all of the ingredients on hand. Keeping a stock of prawns or fish in the freezer can help you on those nights when cooking seems a chore. Rather than reaching for a takeaway menu, whip this simple yet delicious salad up.

Serves 1

25g (0.8oz) soba noodles
6 raw prawn cutlets
4 asparagus spears
½ small red capsicum (pepper)
1 spring onion (scallion)
1 garlic clove
Wedge of lime
Salt and pepper to taste

1. Place noodles in a small bowl and pour over boiling water according to package instructions. After soaking for several minutes, drain and set aside.
2. Shave asparagus spears or finely slice, along with the red capsicum and spring onion.
3. Add a small amount of olive oil to a hot frying or stir-fry pan before cooking garlic and the prawns until pink in colour. Add asparagus, capsicum and spring onion and stir-fry for a few minutes until just tender. Season with salt and pepper if desired.
4. Add the noodles to the pan and mix through before serving with lemon juice squeezed over the top.

Mains

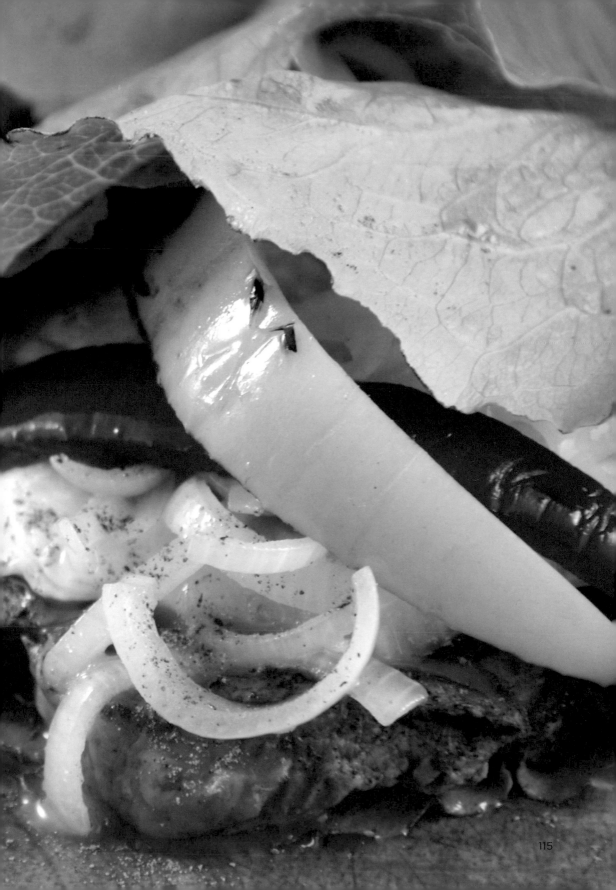

Steak sandwich wraps

A traditional steak sandwich comes with two thick slices of crunchy bread, which is delicious as a sometimes meal but for the other times you want to enjoy a rare steak with a lovely fried egg and some caramelised onions, try substituting lettuce or other large leafy greens in place of bread.

Serves 2

2 x 200g (7oz) scotch fillet steak
2 large lettuce leaves
2 eggs
½ yellow onion
½ red capsicum (pepper)
½ yellow capsicum (pepper)
Salt and pepper to taste

1. Place baking paper over the steaks and use a rolling pin to flatten to desired thickness.
2. Season the steaks with salt and pepper.
3. Heat up a pan or BBQ and cook the steak for a few minutes each side. Leave to rest.
4. Thinly slice the onion and cook in a pan with a drizzle of extra virgin olive oil.
5. Cook the eggs sunny side up in a frying pan.
6. Slice capsicum and roast in the oven at 180°C/356°F for 20 minutes until tender.
7. Assemble the steak sandwich wrap by layering steak, onion, egg and capsicum in a lettuce leaf and rolling.

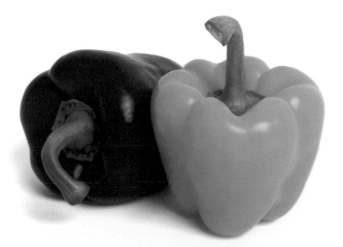

Italian Wedding Soup

There are many variations on an Italian wedding soup, this recipe has a combination of carrots, celery and yellow onion, but you could use whatever vegetables you have on hand in the refrigerator. Traditionally you add chicken or lamb meatballs as well as pasta to bulk the soup up. The meatballs can either be cooked in a pan beforehand or just dropped into the boiling pot, which can save on washing up. The pasta has been omitted in this recipe and replaced with toasted sunflower seeds sprinkled over the top of the soup; they're a great source of magnesium and offer a variation of texture.

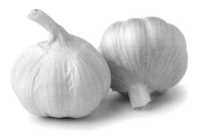

Serves 4

3 carrots, chopped
3 celery stalks, chopped
1 yellow onion, chopped
2 garlic cloves, minced
4 cups (1L) chicken stock
2 cups (500ml) water
1 tbsp dried oregano
250g (8.8oz) chicken mince
½ cup (20g) sunflower seeds

1. Keep the vegetables roughly chopped to add to the rustic nature of the dish. Add the carrots, celery, onion and garlic to a stockpot with a drizzle of olive oil and sweat for 5 – 10 minutes until the vegetables begin to soften.
2. Add chicken stock, water and dried oregano and stir. Simmer over low heat for 30 minutes.
3. Take small handfuls of the chicken mince and roll into balls, keep small so they cook quickly and consistently.
4. Drop chicken meatballs into the soup and stir with a spoon to keep them moving.
5. Take one meatball out after 5 minutes to check it is cooked before removing the pan from the heat and serving.
6. Top the soup with toasted sunflower seeds. Toast the seeds in a dry pan until beginning to brown or in the oven for approximately 15 minutes at 160°C/320°F.

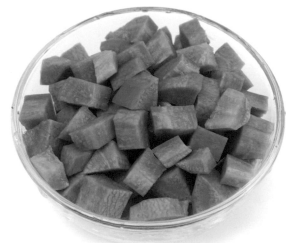

Ricotta gnocchi with zucchini and fennel sauce

There are plenty of substitutes for pasta when you want a lighter option. You can purchase a spiraliser machine or julienne peeler and create vegetable noodles out of most vegetables (zucchini noodles are the most popular). You can also buy spaghetti squash in supermarkets or specialist grocers, which, once cooked, resembles spaghetti noodles. This recipe replaces starchy potatoes in traditional gnocchi with a blend of mostly ricotta and a small amount of flour. Once you've got the hang of making gnocchi it's incredibly easy and these soft little pillows will make you forget all about potatoes.

Serves 2

Ricotta gnocchi
250g (8.9oz) ricotta
1 egg yolk
1 tsp salt
½ cup (55g) plain flour (plus extra for dusting)

1. In a small bowl whisk egg yolk and salt before folding in the ricotta.
2. Using a spoon slowly stir in the flour, being careful not to overwork the mixture.
3. Sprinkle some flour on your work surface and working with a handful of the dough at a time, gently roll starting from the middle and working out until you have a long sausage. If the mixture gets stuck on the work surface simply sprinkle a little more flour over it. Use a knife to cut the sausage into small segments and place on a tray or board lined with baking paper. Repeat with the remaining dough.

Zucchini and fennel sauce
1 large zucchini
½ a bulb of fennel
30g (1oz) butter, cubed
1 tsp ground paprika
1 tsp ground nutmeg
Salt and pepper to taste

1. Slice the zucchini and fennel into thin strips.
2. Heat a frying pan and melt the butter before adding the zucchini, fennel, paprika, nutmeg, salt and pepper. Cook until softened.
3. Once the water has come to the boil add the gnocchi and cook until they come to the surface.
4. Remove from the pot with a slotted spoon then add to the frying pan of sauce. Gently stir through the sauce before serving.

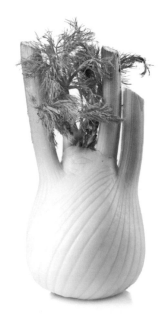

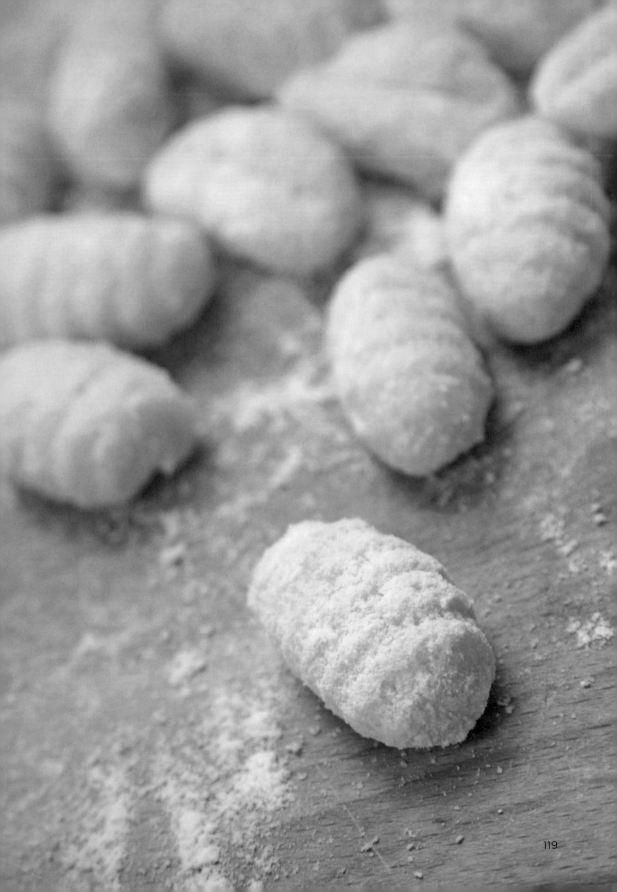

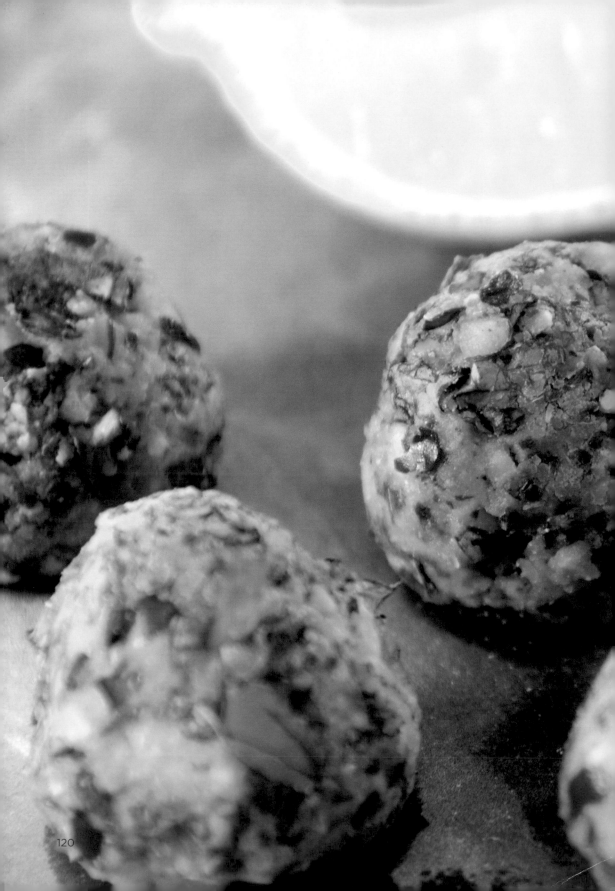

Snacks
and
Sweets

Spicy chickpea & kale bombs

1 cup (400g) chickpeas
1 cup (65g) baby kale
1 tsp ground coriander
1 tbsp chilli flakes
Pinch of sea salt and black pepper
25g (0.8oz) cheddar cheese, grated

1. Pre-heat the oven to 180°C/365°F and line a baking tray with greaseproof paper.
2. Drain chickpeas from tin and rinse under cold water thoroughly.
3. Use a food processor or hand blender to blitz chickpeas, baby kale, coriander, chilli flakes, sea salt and black pepper and mix well.
4. Add grated cheese to the mix and roll into small balls. Dampen your hands with water to help roll the balls if needed. Lay the balls on the baking paper lined oven tray and bake in the oven for 15 – 20 minutes until slightly golden and firm.
5. Store in an airtight container in the refrigerator.

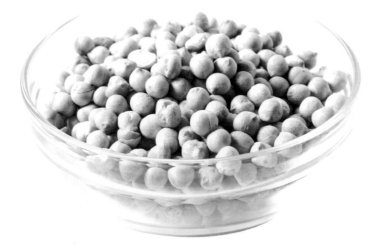

Very Berry Panna Cotta

Panna cotta is a great dessert because you can make it as sweet or tart as you like. This recipe keeps the panna cotta tart and relies on the medley of berries on top to add the desired sweetness. You can use coconut milk, almond milk or even regular milk to customise for dietary needs and flavour. You can sweeten with rice malt syrup or try a small amount of raw honey.

Raw honey that is locally sourced and hasn't been heat-treated has an abundance of healing properties to consider. You won't find this type of honey on your supermarket shelf, anything sitting there has been heat treated and processed to remove all of the beneficial elements and leave only the sweetness. Your local farmer's market is a great source for raw honey, as is the Internet.

Raw honey ensures a premium product that has retained most or all of the beneficial enzymes, natural vitamins and antioxidants. It is anti viral, anti bacterial, promotes good digestive health and can be a powerful aid in treating allergies, particularly hay fever. A little bit goes a long way so you'll find a jar of raw honey will keep you going for many months, if not longer. If you can't source good quality raw honey don't substitute with a supermarket shelf brand, simply avoid it entirely.

1½ cups (375ml) coconut milk
⅓ cup (80ml) rice malt syrup or raw honey
Pinch of vanilla powder
¼ cup (60ml) water
1 tbsp gelatine
1½ cups (405g) Greek yoghurt
Zest of 1 lemon

2 cups (300g) mixed fresh or frozen berries
¼ cup (60ml) lemon juice
1½ tsp cinnamon

1. In a small saucepan heat coconut milk, rice malt syrup and water over a low heat until combined.
2. Sprinkle gelatine over the top of the mixture and stir until dissolved.
3. Remove the pan from the heat and stir through Greek yoghurt and lemon juice.
4. Divide mixture evenly between ramekins or moulds and place in the refrigerator to set for 3 – 4 hours.
5. Macerate berries with lemon juice and cinnamon until soft. Serve each panna cotta with berries poured on top.
6. Panna cottas will keep in the refrigerator for up to two days.

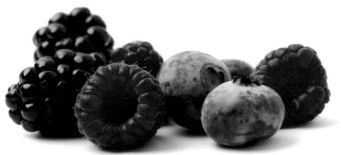

Apples with hazelnut dipping sauce

1 cup (170g) roasted hazelnuts, skins removed
½ cup (40g) shredded coconut
1 cup (250ml) coconut milk
1 – 2 tbsp rice malt syrup (depending on desired sweetness)
1 tbsp raw cacao powder
1 apple

1. In the bowl of a food processor blitz roasted hazelnuts into a fine crumb.
2. Add shredded coconut, coconut milk, rice malt syrup and raw cacao powder. Blitz until smooth and creamy.
3. Slice an apple up into segments and dip into the hazelnut sauce. Store the sauce in an airtight container in the refrigerator.

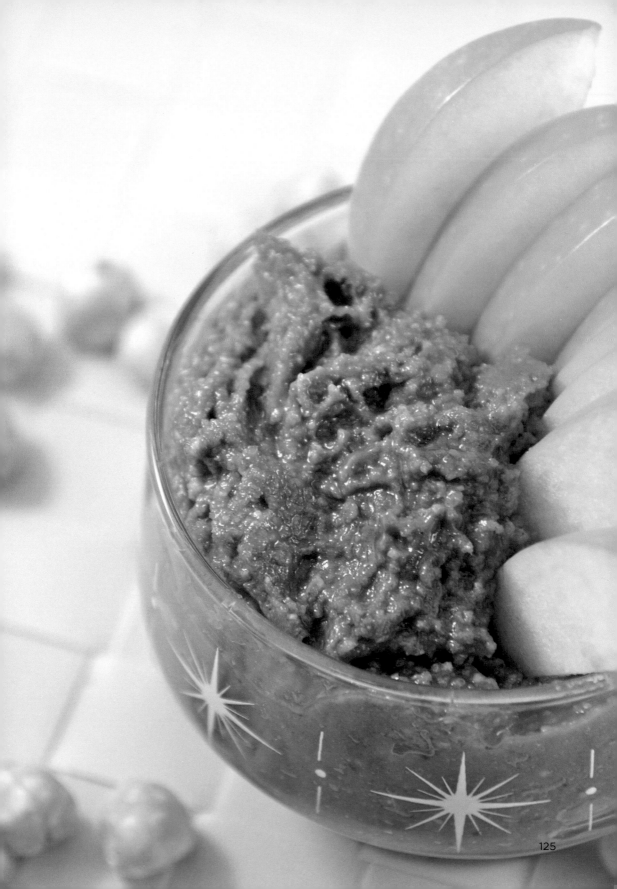

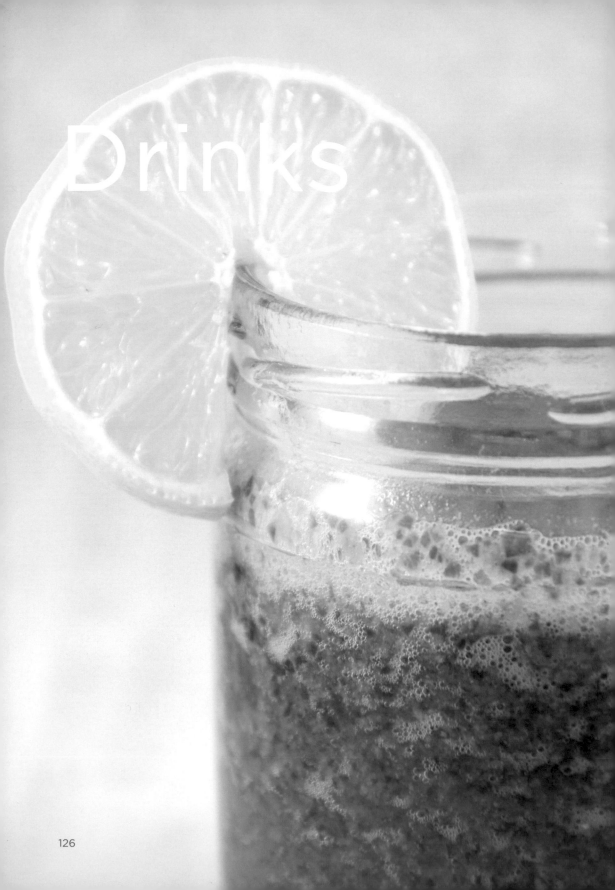

Drinks

Iced Chai Tea

Many iced chai teas or coffees call for using concentrated chai syrup, which can be lovely when you have all the ingredients on hand. This simple iced chai tea uses chai tea bags, which contain most of the spices you'll need. It's super simple and delicious, perfect warm or chilled with plenty of ice.

1 chai tea bags
3 – 4 cups (750ml-1L) of water
Peel of 1 lemon
¼ cup (60ml) rice malt syrup
1 cup (250ml) water, soda water or almond milk

1. In a small saucepan, place tea bags, water and lemon peel and bring to the boil.
2. Reduce to a simmer, remove the tea bags using tongs or a slotted spoon and stir through the rice malt syrup to desired sweetness.
3. Take off the heat and let cool to room temperature before pouring into a jar or jug and chilling in the refrigerator for at least 30 minutes.
4. To serve, fill each glass with ice cubes, pour over the tea mixture to half way up the glass and top with water, soda water, almond milk or the milk of your choice.

Green breakfast smoothie

This recipe is not only loaded with nutritious greens but it's a quick and easy meal on the go for those racing out the door in the morning or needing a quick pick-me-up. If you're worried a smoothie won't fill you up or keep you going all morning, serve alongside an egg on a piece of wholegrain toast, but try it first, you might be surprised!

1 cup (67g) baby spinach (or kale, silver beet)
1 ripe banana (frozen for extra creaminess)
½ an avocado
1 small Lebanese cucumber
½-inch piece of fresh ginger root
1½ cups (375ml) water (almond milk or coconut water)
¼ cup (60ml) lemon juice (fresh)
Pinch of cinnamon
Handful of ice

1. Chop all ingredients up into similar sized chunks.
2. Combine spinach, banana, avocado, cucumber, ginger, water, lemon juice, cinnamon and ice in a blender and blend on high until smooth and creamy.
3. If more liquid is needed add in additional water a little at a time until desired consistency is reached.

Index

For further information

Anyone interested in more information on diabetes prevention and management should use materials produced or recommended by the following organisations or their affiliates in other countries:

International Diabetes Federation
www.idf.org

American Diabetes Association
www.diabetes.org

Diabetes UK
www.diabetes.org.uk

Diabetes Australia
www.diabetesaustralia.com.au

Diabetes New Zealand
www.diabetes.org.nz